GUT instincts

For Alexander and Lilly,
watching you grow is a joy.

GUT
instincts

A **practical guide** to a
healthy digestive system

DR ANDREW BRETT & ANDREA CARSON

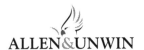
ALLEN&UNWIN

First published in 2007

Allen & Unwin
83 Alexander Street
Crows Nest NSW 2065
Australia
Phone: (61 2) 8425 0100
Fax: (61 2) 9906 2218
Email: info@allenandunwin.com
Web: www.allenandunwin.com

National Library of Australia
Cataloguing-in-Publication entry:

Carson, Andrea.
  Gut instincts.

  Includes index.
  ISBN 978 1 74175 094 2 (pbk.)

  1. Irritable colon - Popular works. I. Brett, Andrew. II.
  Title.

616.342

Set in 11.5/14 pt Adobe Garamond by Midland Typesetters, Australia
Printed and bound in Australia by Griffin Press

10 9 8 7 6 5 4 3 2 1

Contents

List of figures

Acknowledgements

This book would not have been possible without the help, guidance and expert opinion from good friends, colleagues and dedicated professionals. We are also grateful to the many patients who have shared their stories. We would like to sincerely thank Dr Sandra Ray for her patience and advice checking medical facts, reading and re-reading chapters, and encouraging us every step of the way. Thanks also to Professor Peter Gibson, who despite being an extremely busy, internationally esteemed gastroenterologist, kindly found the time to write the foreword to this book. Professor Gibson has been a great source of inspiration to Andrew because of his care for patients and dedication to researching and teaching gastroenterology. A heartfelt thanks also to Sue Shepherd at the Box Hill Hospital for giving her time to check this book and for generously helping us to better understand nutrition and diet, particularly in relation to irritable bowel syndrome and coeliac disease. No book with information about stomal care would be complete without the guidance of clinical nurse specialist Rae Bourke from the Royal Melbourne Hospital. Thank you Rae for your time and advice. As well, thanks to Mike Purvus, also at the Royal Melbourne Hospital, who kindly sourced many of the medical images for this book. Thank you also to Edgar Jaramillo at www.gastrosource.com for allowing us permission to use his medical photographs and to Madeleine Brett for her artistic skills and time.

We would also like to thank our agent Lyn Tranter for her encouragement and professional guidance in the world of publishing, and Annette Barlow at Allen & Unwin for her enthusiasm and faith in this book. Also, to our editors Alexandra Nahlous and Susin Chow for their meticulous efforts putting the book into shape, we are truly grateful; thank you to Ian Faulkner for his great illustrations. We are also indebted to Barbara Alysen at the University of Sydney for her friendship and support, not to mention for also teaching Andrea much of what she knows about journalism. Finally, thank you to Amy Livingstone for looking after our treasures Alexander and Lilly, and to our families and friends for their love and support.

Foreword

Professor Peter Gibson,
Professor of Medicine, Monash University,
Boxhill Hospital, and Director of Medicine and
Gastroenterology, Eastern Health, Melbourne

The gastrointestinal tract (more simply known as the 'gut') constantly reminds us of its presence. Most other organs in the body, such as the heart and lungs, function most of the time beyond our consciousness. In contrast, every time we put food or drink into our mouths or expel waste material of gaseous or solid nature we are aware of its function or dysfunction. It seems improper then that the gut takes a lowly place in our everyday talk or in dinner party conversation. It is not unusual to hear talk of someone's heart attack, arthritis or broken bones, but not about their diarrhoeal illness, Crohn's disease or malodorous expulsions! In contrast, the gut figures prominently in the more seedy side of conversation, where vomiting, defecating (or more specifically its products) and farting (if you can find a better word for it, please let us know) play a prominent place in 'toilet humour' or other unpleasantries. Yet eating is one of the most social and enjoyable things we do in life, and having a satisfying bowel motion leaves one with a feeling of pleasure and peace (why else would 'high colonic irrigation' become popular?).

Why would I choose the less glamorous career path of gastroenterology, where aspects of medicine such as abdominal complaints and bowel function are my bread and butter? After all, I could not claim a record of good tolerance to bodily excrement of others as a child, or even as an adult! Was it that I was a masochist or was it because the gastrointestinal tract is the most diverse, most fascinating and arguably most important part of our body? Opinions vary on this question, but I tend not to view myself as masochistic.

During more than 30 years of clinical and academic gastro-enterology, I have been constantly amazed at the profusion of ideas and hypotheses about the causes and meaning of gastrointestinal symptoms. Libraries and bookstores are full of tomes outlining theories and solutions for many real and some uncertain conditions. For example, we used to have many books on why peptic ulcers formed. These books often centred on stress, the modern world and how we eat. Most of those have been retired to the book graveyard now that Australians, Robin Warren and Barry Marshall, have discovered the real cause—a simple infection with a bacterium called helicobacter—and cure for most ulcers in their Nobel-prize winning work. There is now a profusion of books on how to fix irritable bowel syndrome. It is not difficult to see why, since conservative medicine has so far not had a good record of finding solutions for this common problem. Invariably, the hypotheses in these books are backed up by scientific 'facts' which usually sound feasible when used out of context in a setting that is marketing an idea. Some people have called this 'pseudoscience'. Sometimes the theories or the solutions are or prove to be valid, but it is extraordinarily difficult for the non-expert to differentiate beautifully crafted fiction from fact.

So why has this book been written and why is it so important? Gut complaints are so common. Irritable bowel syndrome may affect up to one in five of us, bowel cancer affects up to one in twelve and coeliac disease might be present in one in a hundred. Most of us will have experienced a bout of diarrhoea, some indigestion after grandma's pastries, or the occasional need to reach for the prunes or the pharmacist's treasure chest of laxatives for constipation. In other words, gut symptoms make up a normal part of our existence. The distinction between normal and abnormal is indeed blurred and can sometimes be challenging even for the experienced health professional. How hard is it then for the untrained observer or sufferer? We all need some guidance in this area, some source of unbiased information that is reliable, easy to understand and free from pseudoscience. We need help in differentiating minor complaints that are effectively part of being normal from symptoms that might potentially point to serious illness.

The work of an enthusiastic, young and highly regarded physician and gastroenterologist, this book is designed to put the myths in their place, and to provide a resource of information that is balanced, accurate and trustworthy. The work avoids pet theories and much of the nonsense that contaminates other books on the gut. It is designed to encourage people with abdominal complaints to appropriately seek help from their family practitioner. The book will be helpful for those trying to understand or put into perspective the illnesses of loved ones or friends. It also provides important information on where to go for further information on specific issues. Overall, it should prove to be an important addition to many people's personal library, where it will help individuals to a greater understanding of abdominal symptoms, the gastrointestinal tract and diseases that affect it.

Introduction

For many of us, there are few greater pleasures that we can regularly indulge in other than eating and drinking. Food is vital to our health, important to our psychological wellbeing and a wonderful way to share, socialise and learn about other cultures and traditions. Preparing and cooking food can also be fun.

So when things go wrong with our digestive system, it is very upsetting. It can be detrimental to our health, lifestyle and happiness. Also, changes to one family member's diet can affect the meal routine of the whole family. Yet, despite the obvious importance of being able to eat and enjoy food, our digestive tract is often something we take for granted until things go wrong.

For many people, the digestive system is a cause of embarrassment. It can make unwanted gurgling and farting noises, and just talking about digestive problems, from bad breath to itchy bottoms or more serious conditions such as blood in our stools, can be uncomfortable for us. So, even when something does go wrong, we often prefer to ignore it rather than get help. But ignoring the problem can be dangerous to our health. At worst, treatable problems can develop into life-threatening conditions.

Well, be embarrassed no longer. Most Australians experience digestive problems at some stage in their lives. Many sufferers are quite young—in their mid-twenties or less. In my clinical practice I have treated patients as young as fourteen with serious disease. Gastrointestinal problems—or tummy troubles—can affect any one of us and they are the most common complaint seen by general practitioners (GPs). Many famous people have suffered gastrointestinal problems: among them are politicians such as John F. Kennedy, who suffered colitis; the French emperor, Napoleon Bonaparte, who died from a perforated stomach ulcer; the 34th President of the United States Dwight D. Eisenhower had Crohn's disease; and George W. Bush recently had a colonoscopy to rule out bowel cancer. Entertainers such as the pop singer Anastacia and Mike McCready, the guitarist of the American rock band Pearl Jam, have spoken publically about having Crohn's disease.

An estimated 40 per cent of Australians have lower gut disorders. One in five Australians is known to suffer from irritable bowel syndrome (IBS) according to the Gastroenterological Society of Australia. But because many sufferers are too embarrassed to see their doctor, many more Australians are thought to be suffering the condition in silence.

What's more, digestive disorders are on the increase. This is particularly evident among busy people under pressure, including, from my clinical experience, many second-generation Australians who feel great pressure to perform, particularly given the sacrifices their parents have made for them to afford their modern lifestyles.

This book aims to help *you* improve your digestive health by better understanding digestive problems and how to treat them. In these pages we freely discuss all types of disorders from the minor to the serious, and talk about what you can expect from the doctor and other health practitioners when things go wrong. There are many things that people with digestive problems can do to help their condition. This includes non-medical therapies such as changing lifestyle to reduce stress, changing diets to improve digestion and removing foods that may irritate the gut. You may not be aware, but new research indicates that intolerances to some fruit sugars may make IBS worse in some people. Depending on your individual situation, alternative therapies, such as massage or relaxation exercises, and medical treatments such as drugs may be of help to you. This book is designed to give you the knowledge to make the necessary changes to improve your digestive health. Or, if you have a family member or friend with digestive disorders, these pages will help you understand what your loved one may be experiencing and why. We aim to look at these problems from your point of view, using easy-to-understand language, with accurate and up-to-date medical information. For this reason, we have added a resource section where you can find further help in the form of self-help groups, specialist medical centres, support organisations, useful websites and further recommended reading.

A selection of recipes has also been included for the conditions where diet plays a key role to get you started on a healthy eating plan. These recipes use foods that soothe the bowel rather than irritate it. The choices vary to cater for digestive needs, ranging from gluten intolerance to inadequate fibre intake, lactose intolerance and more.

But first, a quick word about the language we use to describe the digestive system and what the system is. It is a marvellous labyrinth that takes in food and drink, absorbs vital nutrients and sends them around our bodies to nourish our cells and repair damaged tissue, and then expels what we don't need. It is a complex network of organs, glands, muscles, nerves and chemicals that interacts with our lymphatic, circulatory and nervous systems to feed and water our body. This book is primarily focused on the gastrointestinal tract, the pipe work that extends from the mouth to the anus. Sometimes it is referred to as the GIT, which should not be confused with the *gut*. The gut generally refers more specifically to our intestines, although some people use gut to mean anything to do with digestion. This book uses GIT when referring to the whole or any part of the gastrointestinal system.

In the first chapter, we will take you on a tour of the GIT including the anatomical features of the system, how it works and why it is so important to our health. Chapter two looks in detail at what you can expect from your doctor and other health professionals, beginning with the first visit. In chapter three, we look at common GIT complaints that we all experience from time to time and we clear up some popular myths and misunderstandings about these conditions, including burping, reflux, diarrhoea, constipation, loss of appetite, hiccups and more. We also look at the major symptom of many GIT complaints—abdominal pain—and discuss what it is, what it feels like and what it can mean.

In chapter four, we begin our chapter-by-chapter discussion of more serious GIT disorders. Dedicating a chapter to each topic, we discuss irritable bowel syndrome; peptic ulcers; gastro-intestinal reflux disease (GERD); coeliac disease; inflammatory bowel diseases (IBD), including Crohn's disease and ulcerative colitis; and diverticulitis. Each chapter looks in detail at what the disorder is, who it can affect, what the symptoms are, how it can be treated, what you can do to help with your treatment, what the prognosis is, and what you can expect from your doctor. Each chapter also has case studies and answers to commonly asked questions.

Chapters ten and eleven are about getting help. Chapter ten is concerned with non-drug treatments, particularly alternative therapies and lifestyle changes. Chapter eleven is dedicated to stoma therapy, where to get help and how to live a full life with a stoma.

Lastly, and importantly, this book looks at the effects a gastrointestinal illness can have on our lives and the measures we can take to prevent further episodes of illness. We discuss future treatments that are likely to be available, and say a few words on the latest research. We hope this book will lift some of the myths about our gut and its function. Most importantly, we hope this book helps you to improve your digestive health and to enjoy life's wonderful pleasures of eating, drinking and socialising.

1
The digestive system:
How it works

What is the gastrointestinal tract (GIT)?

The simplest way to describe the GIT is as a pipe that extends from the mouth to the anus.

The GIT is 8 to 9 metres long, and comprises the mouth, oesophagus (gullet), stomach, small intestine (small bowel), large intestine (colon), rectum (back passage), anal canal and anus. The small and large intestines are collectively known as the bowel, and also as the gut.

The tract is a continuous muscular tube and has an enormous blood and nerve supply. It is thought that almost half of our blood (40 per cent) runs through our digestive system after eating a meal. It needs this huge blood supply to carry nutrients from the digestive system to the rest of the body. This is also why some people advise that you should not exercise *immediately* after a big meal, because blood is needed to help with digestion, rather than being diverted away to muscles in the arms and legs as it is during exercise.

The main job of the GIT is to take food and drink and break it down into useable components so that the body can absorb and use them for energy. Energy is needed for all bodily functions including growth, repair and maintenance of the cells that make up our organs, tissue, bones, skin and so on.

The GIT is also responsible for the removal of solid waste from the body in the form of faeces. As you will see, each section of the GIT has a special role in the various breakdown, digestion, absorption and elimination processes.

Figure 1.1 The gastrointestinal tract (GIT) extends from the mouth to the anus

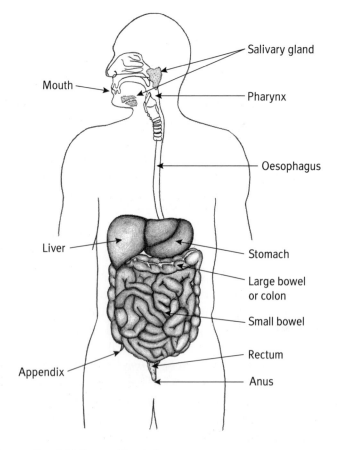

Source: Royal Melbourne Hospital

Mouth

Digestion begins in the mouth after our senses alert us to food. It is both mechanical and chemical. The mechanical part is our teeth chomping and breaking the food into smaller bits to make swallowing easier. The chemical part is one reason why we have saliva (spit); another is that saliva helps lubricate food to make it easier to swallow. It is produced by the salivary glands. We have three sets of salivary glands that open into the mouth: the parotid, the submandibular (which produces most of our saliva), and the sublingual. Saliva contains the enzyme amylase (sometimes called ptyalin). Our senses, such as sight, smell, taste and even the thought of food, stimulate the salivary glands to make saliva. They also stimulate the stomach to produce gastric secretions in readiness for food. We make about 1.5 litres of this slightly acidic fluid (or gastric secretions) every day. Once food is in our mouths, amylase breaks down the carbohydrate component in our food by reducing starch into more basic sugars.

While there is not a set number of times that each mouthful should be chewed, it is important to chew enough times to make food pieces small so they do not get lodged in the oesophagus, and so that enzymes can penetrate the food mass.

Connecting the mouth to the oesophagus is the throat or pharynx. Near the pharynx is an area of muscle known as the **upper oesophageal sphincter** (UOS). The UOS helps with swallowing and stops air going down the oesophagus.

Oesophagus

This thin muscular pipe, sometimes called the food pipe or gullet, transports drink and chewed food from the mouth to the stomach, where further breakdown of food occurs. The oesophagus is about 25 cm long. It pushes food towards the stomach by contracting the muscles and creating a wave-like motion called **peristalsis**. The contractions are strong, even strong enough to defy gravity if you happen to eat or drink lying down or upside-down (though obviously this is in no way recommended!).

Lower oesophageal sphincter

At the end of the oesophagus and the opening of the stomach is a valve called the **lower oesophageal sphincter** (LOS). It is a ring of muscle that acts as a gate and opens to let food into the stomach and, when it is working properly, closes to stop food in the stomach moving back into the oesophagus. A loose LOS allows acidic stomach contents back into the oesophagus: this is called **reflux**, and is discussed in chapter six.

Diaphragm

The diaphragm, a band of muscles below the lungs that helps us breathe, also helps keep the contents of the stomach from coming up the oesophagus by helping to keep the LOS shut. Sometimes, especially in overweight and pregnant people, the stomach slides above the diaphragm, which can make reflux worse. This is called a **hiatus hernia** (and is discussed in chapter six).

Stomach

The stomach is a J-shaped muscular bag that holds ingested food and works like a washing machine by mechanically and chemi-cally mixing the partially digested contents. It has three parts —the **fundus**, the **body** and the **antrum**. The first two are specialised for storage of food, while the antrum is specialised for mixing the food. The stomach is also very flexible—in a baby, it holds about 30 ml, and up to 2 litres in an adult. It has very thick muscular walls covered in about 3 mm of mucus. The mucus protects the stomach from highly acidic juices that the stomach releases to further break down food. These juices are produced in the antrum of the stomach. They are made up of hydrochloric acid and a small amount of protease, an enzyme that breaks down protein. While the acid protects us from bacteria and other bugs that we ingest, too much acid or not enough mucus can lead to holes in the stomach wall—ulcers. Often, this can be caused by an infection from bacteria called *Helicobacter pylori.* (See chapter five on peptic ulcers for more information.)

Figure 1.2 The stomach and intestines

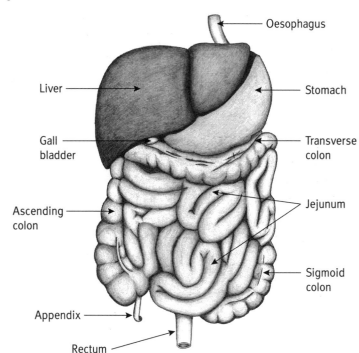

Oesophagus

Liver

Stomach

Gall bladder

Transverse colon

Ascending colon

Jejunum

Sigmoid colon

Appendix

Rectum

Source: Royal Melbourne Hospital

The stomach's muscular lining has ridges that contract to churn the food around and help it to mix with the gastric juices—like a washing machine. We have few sensory nerves in this part of our body, so thankfully the stomach can do its job without us being too aware of it, although occasionally we can feel and hear our stomach grumbling.

After several hours, when the food has been further reduced in size and mixed with the gastric secretions, the contents gradually pass into the small intestine where further digestion and most of the nutrient absorption takes place. A sphincter called the **pylorus** acts as a valve between the end of the stomach and the beginning of the small intestine. It controls the release of contents into the small intestine. The rate at which food enters the small intestine depends on the calorie content of meals; on average, the human stomach delivers about 628 kJ per hour (or 150 Cal/hr). At this point the food looks like broth and is called **chyme**.

Some things are absorbed in the stomach and into the bloodstream, such as drugs and fluids, including water and a small amount of alcohol. This is why thirst is quickly quenched upon drinking and the effects of alcohol and drugs can be felt soon after being taken. However, alcohol is generally absorbed in the small bowel, and having a full stomach can slow down the rate at which alcohol is delivered to the small bowel, which is why it can be a good idea to have something to eat before drinking alcohol.

Small intestine

In a newborn, the small intestine, or small bowel, starts at about 2 metres long and grows to about 6 metres in an adult (three times the height of the child or adult). It can vary a little from person to person and be between 4 and 7 metres. It loops like a series of stretched S-shaped curves inside the abdomen. Unlike the acidic stomach, the small intestine provides an alkaline environment to protect it from the acidic chyme.

The small intestine's key role is to absorb nutrients. Because of this it has been designed to have the maximum amount of surface area for its length. It does this through having **villi**, tiny finger-like projections that stick out of the bowel wall, and **microvilli**, even smaller fingers that stick out of each villus. Each villus is about 1 mm tall. A single villus houses thousands of microvilli. Together, they dramatically increase the surface area of the small intestine, making it 600 times larger—in fact the surface area of the small bowel is bigger than a tennis court! The small intestine has an average width of 4 cm and is made up of three sections: the duodenum (about 30 cm long), the jejunum (2 to 3 metres, or about 40 per cent), and the ileum (3 to 4 metres, about 55 per cent). Most books and references vary in the lengths quoted for these three sections of small intestine because they can differ. The jejunum feels thicker than the ileum to the surgeon when handled, but there is no visible anatomical difference distinguishing the two sections. The ileum connects with the large intestine. The small bowel also contains lymphoid tissue (immunity cells) to fight micro-organisms and bacteria that can harm the body. Chyme is pushed through the small intestine by peristalsis, the same wave-like motion that occurs in the oesophagus and stomach.

Duodenum

The duodenum is the first section of the small bowel and connects the stomach to the jejunum. It is a C-shaped loop that coils around the head of the pancreas. In the adult, the length of the duodenum is approximately 30 cm (or 12 inches, hence its name duodenum—two plus ten). This first segment of the small intestine absorbs important minerals used to build and repair cells such as calcium (bone), iron (blood) and zinc (skin). It also contains the opening of the bile duct and the duct carrying secretions from the pancreas.

It is through the bile duct that a thick, yellow-greenish fluid called **bile** is released into the duodenum. It is released from the gall bladder, but made in the liver. Much the same way as dishwashing detergent emulsifies the fat off our pots and pans, bile breaks down fat into its components, called fatty acids and glycerin, ready for the body to use. The liver sends bile for storage to the gall bladder. When needed, the gall bladder contracts and releases bile into the duodenum via the bile duct. Both the duct and gall bladder can be blocked by gall stones or, more rarely, tumours, and in more severe cases may need to be removed. If the gall bladder is removed, bile runs directly from the liver to the duodenum.

One of the main jobs of the pancreas is to produce enzymes that break down food components into a form which the bowel can absorb. These enzymes include: **amylase**, which breaks down carbohydrate; **proteases** that help digest proteins; and **lipase**, which acts on fat. These are all released into the duodenum.

Jejunum

The jejunum is between 2 and 3 metres long and is where most of the nutrients are absorbed through the villi. It also absorbs most of our ingested fat once the bile has emulsified it. The presence of dietary fibre can reduce the rate of absorption of nutrients here.

Ileum

This part of the small intestine continues to absorb nutrients, but not as many. The villi are slightly smaller and their main job is to absorb water and salts. Bile salts excreted from the liver are also reabsorbed here and reused. The last part of this 3 to 4 metre pipe is also the area where vitamin B12 is absorbed, which is an essential element for blood production. The ileum has more lymphoid tissue, disease-fighting cells, than other parts of the small intestine.

Large intestine

The large intestine, or colon, is about 1 metre long in the adult (about 30 to 40 cm at birth) and is curved like an upside-down U-shape. It is connected to the ileum of the small intestine by the **ileo-caecal valve**. This valve controls the flow of chyme into the large bowel and stops the bacteria-rich environment of the large bowel from flowing back into the relatively clean small bowel.

The large intestine has several parts: the caecum at the beginning of the large bowel, the ascending colon, the transverse colon, the descending colon (and the narrowest section), the sigmoid colon, followed by the rectum and anal canal.

The appendix hangs down from the caecum and is considered redundant in the modern human. The appendix is thought to have played a role in digesting plant material when humans had a different diet to today.

Most of the digestion and absorption of nutrients has occurred by the time they reach the colon. The passage of matter slows down in the colon and takes between twelve and 48 hours to complete. The job of the colon is mainly to absorb water and salt and store the waste products ready for expulsion.

Each day, about 200 to 400 ml of food waste is excreted as faeces. But, if we are dehydrated, the colon can absorb up to five times as much water. This can save us from dying of dehydration in extreme circumstances.

Sometimes, for myriad reasons—drugs, exercise and so on—the food waste in the bowel can move too fast and less water is absorbed resulting in diarrhoea. Conversely, if food residue moves too slowly, more water is absorbed and we can become constipated.

Compared to the small intestine, the contents of the colon has a billion more bacteria per gram and also several hundred different species more than in the small intestine. This is because gut motility, gastric acid and the ileo-caecal valve stop the bacteria in the small intestine reaching the same numbers as in the colon. Also, some of the bacteria play a useful role in the large intestine. They metabolise some fibre, and unabsorbed lipids, proteins and carbohydrates. Normal bowel bacteria also play a role in metabolising some drugs, cholesterol and hormones. Some of the good bacteria also make vitamin K, an important ingredient in blood clotting. Bacteria can be harmful if they enter the bloodstream, but to guard against this the bowel walls are covered in a mucous film to keep the bacteria in the colon.

The leftover waste, made up of water, bile pigments, undigested fibre and spent bacteria, is stored in the rectum then passes through the anal canal where it is excreted out of the body through the anus. Internal and external anal sphincters are two valves that help to control the timing of the passage of the faeces.

We only have conscious control over the external sphincter so that we don't get caught needing to go to the toilet at an inconvenient time. When it is time, stretch receptors in the rectum send a signal to the brain giving us the urge to go to the toilet. Depending on our situation, we can choose to suppress the urge, which readjusts the stretch receptors until a more convenient time, or act on it and allow the faeces to pass with the help of muscle contractions.

How often we go to the toilet depends on factors such as what we eat, how much we consume and drink, exercise, medications, how often we sleep and if we are under stress.

Nutrition and the GIT

The digestive tract works to chemically alter the foods we ingest into nutrients so that our body can use them. The three major types of nutrients, called **macronutrients**, are protein, fat and carbohydrates. The body also needs **micronutrients**, which include minerals and vitamins, although these have no calorie content. Macronutrients provide the body with energy, but are also used as building materials (protein), immediate energy (carbohydrates and fats) and stored energy (fats, sometimes carbohydrates). Adults on a normal diet—about 8370 kJ (2000 Cal)—absorb about 95 per cent of ingested nutrients. In Western societies, carbohydrates account for about 45 per cent of our daily food intake. This includes fruit and vegetables, cereals, processed foods, sugar and milk.

Carbohydrates are broken down and absorbed first, then proteins and lastly fats. People tend to feel fuller after eating a fatty meal because fat slows down the rate at which the stomach empties. In Western societies, about 40 per cent of adult energy requirements come from fats—animal (two-thirds of our fat intake) and vegetable (one-third)—which are broken down into fatty acids and glycerin.

Protein accounts for about 10 to 15 per cent of the average Western diet. Dietary proteins are the major source of amino acids and are needed for muscle and tissue growth and repair. We tend to eat more protein than we need to—the average adult only needs about 0.75 grams of protein for each kilogram of body weight—especially with fad diets calling for a reduction in fat or carbohydrates.

The following table shows the amount of energy these basic nutrient components provide when absorbed and metabolised by the body.

Table 1.1 How much energy macronutrients yield

Nutrient	Energy content unit (kJ)	Examples of nutrient-rich food
Protein	17	Meat, fish, eggs, poultry, dairy products, soy
Fat	38	Oil, butter, margarine, nuts, some meats, eggs, dairy products
Carbohydrate	17	Flour, bread, rice, fruit, pasta, potatoes, lollies and sugar
Alcohol	21	Beer, wine, spirits

*Note: 4.184 kJ = 1 Calorie (Cal) = 1 kilocalorie (kcal) = 1000 Calories (Cal). Numbers have been rounded up. The adult person requires on average 8370 kJ (2000 Cal) per day.

When any part of the digestive tract is not working properly, it disturbs our nutritional and fluid intake, which can affect the health of our whole body, including mental and physical function.

A healthy and balanced diet

What is healthy eating? This simple question is obviously not so easy to answer judging by the problems of obesity in Western societies. But, in short, healthy eating is eating from the different food groups to get the vitamins, minerals and energy you need to allow the body to repair itself, to keep bones, teeth and organs healthy, to enable you to do the activities you want to do, to enhance mood and concentration, and to maintain a healthy weight. Broadly speaking, we should aim to eat between 7500 kJ (1800 Cal) and 10 500 kJ (2500 Cal) a day depending on our individual requirements. But, every individual will have different requirements depending on their activities, height, weight, age and sex. If you are worried about your diet or weight, you should see a dietitian to be properly assessed to find a healthy eating program that best suits your individual needs.

As a general guide, you should be getting your kilojoules by eating food from eight different food groups. These are: grains and cereals (four or more serves per day); fruit (two or more serves per day); vegetables (five or more serves per day); meat, fish, chicken and eggs (one to two serves per day); dairy (three serves per day); legumes (two or three serves per week); nuts and seeds (one serve per day); and, lastly, fats (two to three serves per day), aim for polysaturated or monosaturated fats such as those found in olive oil, avocado and nuts. If you imagine these eight groups being squeezed into a pyramid, the largest proportion of our diet should come from unprocessed foods such as fruit and vegetables, nuts, grains and cereals, breads, legumes and beans. These are the base of the pyramid and are what nutritionists recommend we eat most of. These foods should give us most of our energy from complex carbohydrates as well as the vitamins, minerals and dietary fibre that we need. This is where most of our nutrients should come from.

In the middle of the pyramid are foods that we can and should eat, but not excessively. These foods give us the protein we need, as well as minerals, such as iron and calcium, and vitamins. These foods include fish, lean meat (with the fat removed), dairy products, eggs and chicken. This is where some of our nutrients come from.

At the pinnacle of the triangle are the foods we should consume in small amounts each day. They may be tasty but they have fewer nutrients. Foods in this section include fats, sugar and oils. A small intake of fat is not bad for us and will give condition to our hair and skin; in other words, it provides essential fatty acids needed for the production of healthy hair and skin.

As well as these basic principles, you should aim for about 2 litres (about eight glasses) of fluid a day, preferably water; and avoid adding fats and salt to meals. Unless otherwise recommended, you should try to get about 30 grams of fibre a day.

Figure 1.3 How to have a healthy diet

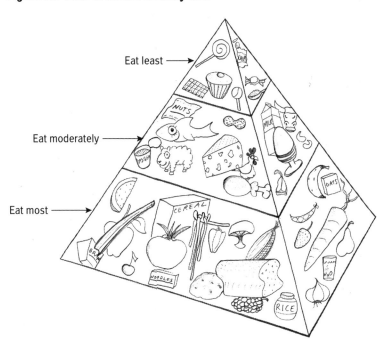

Source: Madeleine Brett

*Note: This illustration is simplistic and does not cater for special dietary needs or vegetarian, vegan or other lifestyle preferences. See a dietitian for more detailed dietary advice.

Hunger

Hunger is a very complex phenomenon that has physical, emotional and psychological triggers. A simple explanation of hunger is that it is a message sent to the brain that tells us to eat. This message can be triggered by our senses—the sight, taste, smell or thought of food—or by our digestive tract. The stomach, which expands and shrinks to accommodate food, has receptors that can tell us when it is stretched. These send a message to the brain to say that we are full. As we all know, there can be a time delay between when the full stomach sends the message to the brain to stop eating, and when we actually do! When the stomach is empty, the receptors trigger another message, which the brain interprets as hunger. Other hunger messages are sent to the brain when our blood sugar level falls and the body needs more energy.

Appetite regulation, which is important to maintain a healthy weight, is believed to involve the interaction of messages in the brain, some coming from the stomach and intestine. Some of the message pathways involve the body releasing hormones, called endorphins and enkephalins, that make you feel good. These chemicals are similar to drugs such as morphine. It is thought these hormones are linked to stress-and-reward triggers, and stimulate eating. Overeating and weight gain can develop when we are stressed. If it is prolonged, the body becomes used to the higher endorphin levels and it is difficult to stop the cycle of overeating.

Fibre

Fibre is the indigestible plant matter found in foods like wholegrain cereals and fruit and vegetables (the skins are a great source of fibre). It can influence how much we eat by slowing down the pace of digestion of food in the stomach and gut. This helps prevent overeating because the extra bulk of fibre stretches the stomach more, and the slowing of food moving through the small bowel sends a message to the brain that we are full. Fibre also regulates the release of sugar into the blood, giving you energy for longer and warding off hunger. The role of fibre and its different types are discussed in more detail in chapter four.

Summary

The main role of the gastrointestinal tract is to absorb water and process food for the body to use. In the mouth, food is broken into smaller pieces and mixed with saliva. Here, carbohydrate digestion has begun. The food is then swallowed and travels down the oesophagus to the stomach. In the acidic stomach, protein digestion begins, and the food is stored until the chyme produced by mixing food with secretions is passed to the small intestine. Here, it is more alkaline and the contents are neutralised so that digestion and absorption of carbohydrates, proteins and fats can occur. The large intestine absorbs water and salts, and stores the leftover material ready for excretion out of the anus. The liver, gall bladder, bile duct and pancreas play important roles in the digestive system by breaking down potentially harmful waste substances and aiding the digestion of food with the release of enzymes, bile and hormones.

A healthy digestive tract is crucial to the adequate nutrient intake which allows us to enjoy good general health. Diet is also important to maintain health. Like a car engine, the kind of fuel used matters to performance. A well-balanced diet and sensible amounts of food eaten at regular meal times will contribute to better health and wellbeing.

2
What to expect at the doctor's clinic

The doctor was pleasant enough to begin with. I was a bit embarrassed describing my symptoms, and probably wasn't very clear. He asked me some questions I didn't expect, like what was my sexual preference. I was put out by that, given I had already told him I was married with two kids. What does that have to do with my abdominal pain and diarrhoea? He said he would write me a referral to see a gastroenterologist, but I didn't go back. Some weeks I still get diarrhoea several times a day, which makes life at work very stressful. I still don't know what is wrong with me but I don't want to go back to the doctor.

John, 38, plumber

When to see the doctor

As John's example above shows, visiting the doctor can be daunting for many of us. Reasons for this include fear of the unknown, embarrassment, a previous bad experience or not wanting to admit to ourselves that we might be unwell. It is easy to make excuses for not making an appointment. We tell ourselves: we are too busy; the doctor won't be able to do anything anyway; it will go away by itself; and there are people a lot sicker than me and they just get on with life. In John's case, his doctor was not helpful because he did not communicate clearly and John was left feeling embarrassed because of it. The important lesson here is—don't give up, find a doctor who you feel comfortable with and who you can talk to easily so that you can get the treatment you need to start feeling better.

For people reading this book who have a gastrointestinal disorder, you should see your doctor when you are feeling unwell and it is interfering with your day-to-day life. Other times for making a doctor's appointment include when:

- Your symptoms get worse.
- You are scheduled for a check-up.
- You are losing weight and unable to put it back on.
- You need your medications reviewed.
- You need to talk to someone about your health and feelings.
- You need further advice and information.

Really, there are no hard rules about seeing the doctor other than **if you have a problem, don't put it off**. If something is worrying you, then it *is* a problem and needs attention. Research has shown that men are more likely to avoid the doctor than women. The Australian Institute of Health and Welfare's annual report found that the Australian population makes more than 90 million visits to general practitioners every year, and most of those visits are by women (nearly 60 per cent). Men aged between fifteen and 44 were the least likely to visit a GP. So, if you are feeling unwell, don't avoid seeing your doctor; even an annual check-up to make sure your blood pressure is okay is worth the visit for the peace of mind.

What to expect: The first visit to a general practitioner

To get the most out of your visit to the GP, you need to do a few things first:

- **Resolve to be honest**—Accept that you must tell your doctor everything, even if it means that you risk feeling embarrassed. It would be hard for your doctor to make the right diagnosis if you withhold important information. If you are talking about bowel problems and you are worried about how to describe it, tell your doctor you are embarrassed. GPs see scores of patients every week and they have heard and seen just about everything. You can be assured that they will not get embarrassed and will not take any offence to the words you use, so tell it like it is.
- **Write things down**—Before you go to your appointment, write down the problems you have been having so you don't forget. Also, make a note of what medications you are on and the dose. Write in your notes if anyone in your family has had the problem before.
- **Consider taking a friend**—If you are worried about cultural or language barriers, or just feel scared, you might want to bring someone with you. Your doctor won't mind. If you have children, it can be hard to concentrate on what the doctor is saying if they are competing for your attention; ask a friend to care for them in the waiting room or at home while you are seeing the doctor.
- **Know what you want**—Before your visit, try and work out what you want from the visit. Do you want to try new medication? Do you want a referral? It helps you and your doctor if you are clear about what you think you need. However, you should not self-diagnose—always listen to your doctor's advice, even if it isn't what you initially wanted.

If you have a lot of questions to ask, be fair to your doctor, who may be pushed for time, and book a double session. You can do this by telling the receptionist at the time of booking that you need extra time this visit.

Once you are at the doctor's clinic, you will tell the receptionist you have arrived. Usually there is a waiting room with some magazines and sometimes children's toys. Try and relax. If you need to, look over your notes so that you are clear about what you want to say.

How the doctor gathers information

Once you are with the doctor, they need to find out some information about you and your symptoms to work out what the problem is. They will take a history, which means asking questions about the immediate problem, and then they will do a physical examination.

Taking a medical history

For your doctor to understand the context of your symptoms, they will need to know some more information about you. This involves asking you questions about your health that might include the foods you eat, your bowel actions and wind or bloating, medications, recent symptoms, recent travel and family medical history. You will be asked if you have experienced any bleeding from the rectum, and to describe your pain in detail and what makes it worse. If it is relevant, you may be asked about your sleep patterns and sex life. Think about the answers to all these questions before your visit, so that you don't miss any important information. If it helps, write down the answers and take them along. Volunteer any information you think might help your doctor understand your problem better.

Usually taking your history involves questions about the immediate problem, then questions about the rest of your health and past medical history. Family medical history is also important. Occupational and recreational activities may also be relevant.

Physical examination

Your doctor will want to do a physical examination. Depending on your symptoms, this might involve listening to your breathing with a stethoscope placed on your bare skin on your back and chest. Some doctors ask you to take off your shirt; others lift up your clothing to put the stethoscope in place. Your doctor will most likely take your blood pressure using a cuff that goes around your upper forearm; and they may check your heart rate by putting their hand on your wrist. For most gastrointestinal problems, they will feel your abdomen and stomach and may want to look in your mouth. Depending on your symptoms, they may need to do a physical examination of the rectum using a gloved, lubricated finger to feel for any abnormalities, a blockage or blood. This involves lying on your side on the examination table and takes no more than a minute or two. It may be uncomfortable but is usually not painful.

The cause of abdominal pain can be hard to diagnose because it can come from any of the organs in the abdomen. Some of these organs share nerve pathways so pain from one organ can appear to be coming from another. For this reason, women with abdominal pain may need a vaginal examination to rule out a gynaecological problem. This takes only five minutes and usually involves your doctor inserting a gloved finger into the vagina and with the other hand pressing gently on the lower abdomen to feel for any abnormalities. Sometimes a plastic or metal instrument called a speculum may be inserted into the vagina to help the doctor get a better look at the cervix. The examination should not be painful, but you may be a little uncomfortable, as you will feel some pushing.

After the physical examination, your doctor might need to gather more information before they can give you a diagnosis. They may order some tests such as a blood test, urine test, X-ray of your stomach or abdomen, and perhaps a CT scan. They may also get you to send in a stool sample to be tested for blood or an infection. Usually these tests involve your doctor giving you a simple referral letter and sending you to a diagnostic centre where the tests will be done, which may or may not be near the doctor's clinic. If you are seeing a doctor in a public hospital, it will all be done at the hospital. Your doctor will then organise to phone you, or for you to come in for another appointment, once the test results are in. In the following section, you will find more information on the individual tests.

If you are not happy with the way you have been treated, or do not feel comfortable with your doctor, see if you can discuss the reasons why with the doctor. They might not realise what you are feeling until you tell them. Sometimes doctors are so busy that they cannot recognise that you need more information. If you are still unhappy, consider changing doctors. It is hard enough coping with an illness without the stress of feeling intimidated or misunderstood by the person whose job it is to help you. It might be worth asking your friends if they can recommend a good doctor. If you want to change doctors, don't be afraid to make the move. Your medical records can easily be transferred to another GP on your request. You need to be able to work with your doctor to solve your medical problems as a team.

From the GP to a specialist: Understanding the doctor referral system

Depending on your symptoms or what the test results are, your GP may want you to see a specialist doctor. These doctors have done extra medical training in a specific area of medicine. For abdominal complaints, the specialist doctor is called a gastro-enterologist. Gastroenterologists are experts on the gastrointestinal system and related organs such as the liver. They are physicians who do not operate, but they do perform diagnostic procedures such as endoscopy (see below).

In Australia, you need your GP to refer you to a gastroenterologist before you can make an appointment. A referral involves your doctor writing a brief letter explaining your medical problems and the reasons why they think you need to see a specialist. Usually, they will give you the letter to take along to your specialist appointment, which you usually book yourself, although some GPs will do it for you. If you do not have private health insurance and are not so unwell as to be in hospital, depending on where you live, you may have to wait up to two months to see a specialist. This is not ideal but in other developed countries, such as the United Kingdom, the waiting times are much longer. If you want to see the specialist more quickly, you can pay to see the gastro-enterologist privately. If you do have private health insurance, you can usually see a specialist within a week. Your GP will usually recommend a particular specialist to you. If you have a preference for someone else, tell your GP and, if it is appropriate, they will be able to refer you to that specialist.

The visit to the specialist will be very similar to seeing a GP, but they may also schedule an endoscopy. If there is an obvious problem, they will see the problem immediately during the proce-dure. Sometimes they may take a small sample of the tissue, called a biopsy, to send to a laboratory to get more information. This procedure is done during the endoscopy and is painless. If the problem is clear-cut, the specialist will explain it to you and advise you on the recommended management. They may want to see you again for a follow-up visit to make sure everything is okay or they may refer you back to your GP for follow-up visits. Either way, the specialist will write a letter back to your GP with their opinion and recommended management of the problem for your GP's records.

Make the most of your visit to the specialist and find out everything you want to know. It is a good idea to write a list of questions before you go, so that you don't forget anything. Examples of some of the questions you might want to ask are at the end of this chapter.

Tests and procedures

Usually doctors will recommend some tests and procedures to be performed to accurately diagnose your symptoms and to arrange appropriate treatment. The common tests and procedures that may be used to diagnose GIT problems are discussed below.

Blood tests

An analysis of the components of your blood and their amounts might be required to help with diagnosis. It is an easy test that takes less than five minutes and feels like a mosquito bite. It involves a nurse or doctor putting a tight band, called a tourniquet, around your upper arm; this raises the blood pressure in your lower arm to make it easier to find a vein. A small needle (attached to a syringe) is then inserted into the vein, usually at the crook of the arm: other veins can be used, but this spot is usually the most convenient. The blood will flow from the needle into the syringe. When enough blood has been taken (up to 20 ml or so), the tourniquet is taken off and the needle is withdrawn quickly to minimise pain. The problems that your doctor is looking for when they send your blood to be analysed are:

- Levels of **iron, vitamin B12** and **folic acid**—Low levels of these can indicate anaemia, which can be a sign of bleeding in the GIT or malabsorption.

- The number of **white blood cells, red blood cells** and **platelets** (the part of the blood that makes it clot)—Altered levels of these can indicate infection, anaemia and many other diseases including, in severe cases, cancer.
- The **inflammation rate** of blood cells—This can be assessed by watching how quickly blood cells sink in a capillary tube, called ESR (erythrocyte sedimentation rate); or another blood test, called CRP (C reactive protein), may be performed. C reactive protein is produced in the liver usually when there is some inflammation present in the body. A high ESR or CRP can indicate infection or the body fighting itself, which happens in auto-immune diseases and inflammatory diseases such as IBD.
- **Liver function**—The enzyme levels in the blood can indicate if the liver is working properly. The liver is involved in many aspects of the body's functions and many diseases can cause it to become inflamed or not function properly, including IBD.
- Special **antibodies**—These are found in the blood when a person has a particular disease such as coeliac disease. It is a very useful diagnostic tool.
- **Calcium** and **phosphate levels**—These can be abnormal if the body is not absorbing or getting enough calcium. Too little calcium can cause bones to become brittle, which is sometimes a problem when insufficient calcium is absorbed because of long-term gastrointestinal illnesses. Magnesium levels may also fall because of malabsorption and diarrhoea. This can lead to symptoms of muscle weakness.

Stool specimens

Taking a stool sample is a simple matter of collecting a small amount of your faeces to be analysed in a laboratory. A stool sample might be checked for:

- **Infection**—The examiner will be looking for a micro-organism that might be causing the diarrhoea.

- **Blood**—This is not always obvious to the naked eye so a solution is added that makes the blood turn blue.
- **Composition**—Sometimes a stool sample is collected over 24 hours to check if too much fat is being excreted. This can indicate a bowel absorption problem or sometimes a liver problem.

Breath tests

This is a simple test, like an alcohol breath test, that involves breathing out while a machine analyses the gas. It is generally used for detecting the presence in the stomach of the bacteria *Helicobacter pylori*, a cause of stomach and intestinal ulcers. A hydrogen breath test can be used to detect fructose malabsorption.

Bowel preparation

For some tests, such as a colonoscopy, or procedures such as bowel surgery, you will need to have a bowel preparation. The reason for this is to make the bowel as empty as possible so your doctor can see what is going on. Bowel preparations may vary a little according to your doctor's preference, but usually involve drinking a clear fluid the night before, and avoiding solid foods. The fluid has a laxative effect, and makes you go to the toilet to empty your bowels. Popular preparations include Glycoprep, Picoprep and Fleet. Don't plan any outings on this night because you may need to have the toilet close by. If your procedure is in the morning, you may also be asked not to eat that morning. Generally, you can have water.

Endoscopies

Endoscopy is a procedure that takes between five and 30 minutes and allows the gastroenterologist to look inside the body. An endoscope is a narrow tube used to look inside the bowel. These scope procedures give the doctor a terrific view of the problem area and make diagnosis easier.

Figure 2.1 A colonoscope

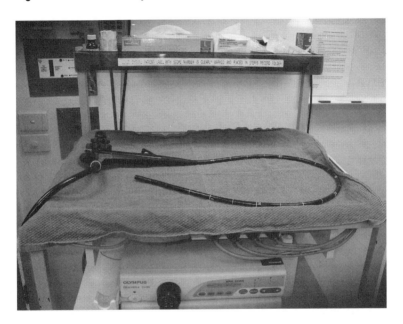

Colonoscopy

Most people these days have a colonoscopy or flexible sigmoid-oscopy. It is the same procedure, but the colonoscopy can travel further up the bowel. Both procedures require a bowel preparation. The doctor or nurse will ask you to lie on your side on a procedure table or bed. A soft, flexible tube, no wider than a finger, with a TV camera and light source at its end, is lubricated and inserted into the bowel via the anus. The procedure takes about ten to 20 minutes. The scope is hollow so that if the doctor needs to do a biopsy of any unusual-looking tissue, it can be taken using a tweezers-like instrument that is inserted into the scope. It shouldn't be painful but you might feel pressure and slight cramping. In Australia, the procedure is done under light sedation and there is usually no memory of the procedure after it is over.

A rigid sigmoidoscope

This is a shorter instrument that does not reach as far as the flexible sigmoidoscope or colonoscope. It goes only about 25 centimetres into the rectum. Its use is more limited and is best for investigating the rectum. A bowel preparation is needed. It is not used very often anymore because colonoscopy gives a better view, and is more comfortable for the patient.

Gastroscopy

A gastroscope is a thin flexible telescopic tube with a tiny light source and camera that goes in the mouth, stomach and first part of the small bowel (duodenum). Gastroscopy takes about five minutes and is usually done under mild sedation. By looking through the tube, or at a TV screen connected to the camera, the doctor is able to check for signs of bleeding, abnormal growths (caused by polyps or tumours), or damage to the inside lining of the GIT (caused by problems such as ulcers or reflux). If something is found, the doctor may take a biopsy to send to the laboratory to investigate further. The patient usually has no memory of the procedure because of the sedation and suffers no pain.

Capsule gastroscopy

This test can be used to look at the small bowel and, more recently, the oesophagus. The patient swallows a tiny pill-sized disposable camera, which sends a video image to a small receiver worn on a belt. The doctor reviews the video later. The camera travels through the bowel and is excreted in the faeces. Although very expensive, this procedure requires no special preparation or an anaesthetic. Its limitation is that no biopsies can be taken.

Proctoscopy

This procedure can be done in the doctor's clinic with no prior preparation. Like the rigid sigmoidoscope it is a short instrument. In this case it only reaches as far as the anal canal and a small part of the rectum and therefore has limited use.

Radiological tests

CT scan (computerised tomography or CAT scan)

This is an advanced type of X-ray that provides an inside view of the body. A special type of CT scan can give pictures similar to a colonoscopy (often called a CT colonoscopy or virtual colonoscopy). It has its limitations (you can't do biopsies) but it is good for detecting abnormalities like cancer and diverticulum. This test requires a bowel preparation the day before.

For a CT scan, you will lie on a table on your side or stomach. The scan is taken by a machine that surrounds the table like a doughnut. The machine takes pictures and the table is able to move through the machine while it quickly takes the images then the computer compiles the information to provide a three-dimensional image of the bowel. You will be in the room by yourself because the machine emits radiation. The level of exposure is safe in small doses, but obviously not for staff who work with the equipment every day. For their protection they will be in an adjoining room, but you will be able to see them through a glass wall or window and you can talk to them through a speaker system. Before leaving the room, your doctor will insert a small, flexible tube into your rectum: This allows air to be gently pumped into the colon using a hand-held squeeze bulb. You will be asked to pump air into the colon to distend it so that the whole of the inside of the bowel can be seen. As the table moves through the scanner, you will be asked to hold your breath for about fifteen seconds. The process is repeated with you lying on your back so that everything is seen. The procedure should take no more than 30 minutes.

Magnetic resonance imaging (MRI) scan

This newly available test provides very clear pictures of the body's organs and tissue by using a magnetic field and radio waves. No X-rays are involved. It is a very safe test, but you are unable to wear anything metal, including jewellery, because of the strong magnetic field. This means that people with pacemakers are unable to have MRI scans. All make-up must be removed because it too can contain metal particles. The procedure involves lying on a table that is inside the machine. It can be daunting at first because it is a tight, enclosed space. If you suffer claustrophobia, you should tell your doctor. The machine will not touch you, but you will hear it buzz and hum as it does its work. The test will take between 30 and 60 minutes, and often you can listen to music during the test. A radiologist will view the images and report the findings back to your doctor within a day or so.

Nuclear medicine scan

Nuclear medicine tests are not used often to diagnose gastro-intestinal disorders because of the quality and ease of the other tests available. The purpose of this test is to locate areas of inflammation. This is done by taking a sample of blood and isolating the white blood cells; these cells fight infection and will be present at any inflamed area in the body. A radioactive component is inserted into the white blood cells and they are then injected back into your body. A gamma camera scans over your body to see where the white blood cells have congregated. Infrequent testing using gamma rays is safe and painless.

Positron emission tomography (PET) scan

PET scans are infrequently used in gastrointestinal medicine. Occasionally they may be ordered if a tumour is suspected. Like the nuclear medicine scan, a PET scan involves inserting a radioactive substance and watching where it goes. In this case, the radioactive marker is added to molecules that are consumed by tumours, such as oxygen and glucose. Tumours grow more quickly than normal tissue, so the radioactive substance should be concentrated around the tumour if one is present.

Bone densitometry (DEXA) scan

Your doctor may want to check the calcium level in your bones if there is the possibility that they are getting thin; this occurs because you have not been absorbing enough calcium from the intestine, or you have been using steroids for some time which affects the absorption of calcium. A bone scan is simple and painless. It involves lying on a table while a machine uses small amounts of radiation to measure the thickness of the bone in the spine and legs (usually the femur). The test usually takes about 30 minutes.

Abdominal X-ray with barium enema

This test is used to get a picture of the inside of the colon. It is not so commonly done in Australia anymore since the use of CT scanning and colonoscopy. However, the barium enema is still useful for seeing inflammation of the bowel, cancer and diverticular disease. A bowel preparation is needed. The actual enema takes around 30 minutes. It involves lying on a table then a lubricated tube is inserted into the rectum. Barium is a non-toxic, white liquid that shows up on X-ray and this is gently poured into the tube into the colon. A small balloon at the tip of the tube stops the barium from flowing out. Sometimes air is puffed into the tube to make the bowel bigger and easier to see inside. The doctor will then take pictures with the X-ray machine which they will be able to see on a TV screen. You need to be still for this so that the pictures are not blurry. In between the pictures, you may need to move from one side to the other so that the barium is coating the entire bowel wall to provide a better image. The procedure can be a little uncomfortable. There can be a feeling of fullness, sometimes some abdominal cramping, and the feeling of wanting to defecate. The tube is removed when enough pictures have been taken. You will probably want to go straight to the toilet or use a bedpan to expel the barium.

Abdominal X-ray with barium meal and barium swallow

This X-ray enables the doctor to have a good look at the stomach and duodenum—the first part of the small intestine. It involves the patient swallowing barium, a non-toxic white chalky-tasting fluid, and then taking an X-ray. The barium fills the stomach and small intestine, and allows the X-ray to make a picture of these structures. It will show if any ulcers or abnormalities are present.

Ultrasound

Also called sonography, this is a method of obtaining images using high-frequency sound waves. The sound waves bounce off the organs and are recorded. Using a computer, the recordings are transferred into images. It is painless and a very safe procedure that does not involve X-rays. It is regularly used in obstetrics to look at the unborn foetus. Unfortunately, it is often not a useful test for assessing the bowel because the ultrasound waves are reflected by gas, and the bowel is often full of gas. But it is good for assessing organs that contain fluid. For this reason, when diverticulitis is suspected, the ultrasound is used to detect pus-filled diverticula.

Diagnosis and prognosis—what do they mean?

Once your doctor has gathered information about you by taking a history, doing a physical examination and interpreting the results of tests and procedures, they will be in a better position to tell you what the cause of the problem is—the **diagnosis**. However, more often than not in medicine, and contrary to most medical dramas on television, the cause or diagnosis remains unclear. This is not as bad as it sounds. Dealing with the symptoms successfully treats many medical problems, even though the underlying cause is not found. Sometimes your doctor may be waiting for a few more signs and symptoms to appear before confirming the diagnosis with you. This is a reasonable thing to do if the diagnosis has a grim outlook, or no cure. For any patient, it is a psychological burden coming to terms with a diagnosis with no cure and no doctor wants a patient to experience that if there is a possibility the diagnosis is wrong.

Prognosis is the word the medical profession uses to describe the long-term 'outlook' of a patient diagnosed with a disease. A prognosis can refer to the quality of life a patient may expect after diagnosis. As we know, not all diseases are curable, but many are treatable and a patient may still have a good quality of life despite having an illness. For example, coeliac disease is not curable but it is treatable. People with coeliac disease who comply with treatment by not eating foods with gluten can live to normal life expectancy and therefore have a very good prognosis. People with coeliac disease who do not change their eating habits and continue to eat food containing gluten will have a shortened life span and therefore have a much poorer prognosis.

The role of surgery

As medical technology advances, surgery is becoming less necessary for many conditions. Despite this, it still occasionally is the best form of treatment, particularly for gall stones and bowel cancer.

Before agreeing to any surgery make sure you are aware of all the risks, benefits and likely outcomes before you come to hospital. If you feel uncertain about anything, ring your doctor and, if still unsatisfied, it may be worth seeking a second medical opinion.

Suggested questions to ask your doctor

Getting the information you need can be hard. Doctors are busy and can talk quickly and assume that you know things you aren't familiar with. Also, when you have been diagnosed with a condition, it is a shock. You may not be able to concentrate on details or absorb information because you are still coming to terms with your illness. This is very normal. Most doctors understand this and will not overload you with information on the first visit, or they may suggest that you bring someone you trust with you, to listen to what is said. Sometimes family members are not a good choice because they are emotionally involved and they too may only hear parts of the messages and get confused. Sometimes other factors get in the way of good communication such as deafness, poor language skills and cultural barriers. If English is not a first language for you, some hospitals offer an interpreter service or pamphlets with easy-to-understand explanations written in other languages. It's always worth asking if these options are available. A good doctor will encourage you to ask questions and to phone their clinic or see them again if you are still unclear about what was said.

There are some practical things you can do before you see your doctor to help you understand your medical condition. Think about the types of things you want to know beforehand. Write them down. Try to be as clear and concise as you can be.

Essentially, most people want to know basic things about their diagnosis, treatment and the prognosis, and how their condition will affect their lifestyle. Some of the most commonly asked questions doctors hear are:

- What is wrong with me?
- What is causing the pain or bleeding?
- Do I need an operation?
- Is it contagious or inherited?
- How long will it last?

- Does it lead to anything more serious such as cancer?
- What do I need to do? Are there changes I need to make to my diet or lifestyle?
- Do I have to give up alcohol?
- What medications do I take? Are there any side effects? Do I have to take them at a certain time of day? How long do I need to be on medication?
- When can I go back to work? Can you write me a medical certificate?
- Can I still do my usual physical activities?
- Will it affect my sex life?
- Can I travel?

Questions to ask before surgery

If you have been told you need an operation, it is crucial that you understand exactly what is going to happen before you sign the consent form. Most doctors, and also the doctor giving the anaesthetic (called an anaesthetist), will take the time to explain the procedure carefully, so that you have realistic expectations about the surgery and quality of life afterwards.

If the operation involves a stay in hospital, you can ask questions of other medical professionals such as your nurse, physiotherapist, surgeon and anaesthetist. Questions to ask may include:

- What will be done? (If relevant, make sure you ask if it involves the left or right side.)
- Will it be an open incision or keyhole surgery (laparoscopic)?
- How will the surgery help?
- If the surgery is more complicated than expected, what other options will the surgeons consider at the time of surgery?
- How long will the operation take?
- What are the possible things that could go wrong?

- What can I expect to see when I wake up from the anaesthetic (i.e. a drip, blood transfusion, a drain tube, bandaged abdomen, catheter to drain urine, etc.)?
- How long will I be in hospital?
- How long does it normally take to recover from this surgery?
- What medications will I need to take?
- Will further follow-up surgery be necessary?

You may want to read about your disease or operation to further your understanding of your situation. Knowledge is power, and learning about your condition is a good idea as long as you choose your source of information wisely and within context. Reading about a very rare side effect can make you feel more anxious than need be. Scaremongering is also a problem when using information available on the Internet. While the Internet is full of information about medical conditions, it is sometimes difficult to verify the accuracy of this information and to apply it appropriately to your situation. Many commercial interests publish selective medical information to try and sell their products and, in the process, truth is compromised. If you want to do further reading, ask your doctor or nurse if they can recommend any good books, websites or support organisations. Many hospitals and doctors' clinics have free pamphlets for patients wanting more information.

Who else can help?

If you have been diagnosed with a chronic disease or you have an illness that has a poor prognosis, you will have good days and bad days as you come to terms with your situation. This is normal and very understandable. It can feel like a lonely experience because your family and friends may want to help you, but do not fully understand what you are going through despite their good intentions.

Most probably there is someone who will understand what you are going through because they have experienced it too, or they have years of professional experience working with people in your situation.

It is a good idea to consider making contact with a support group, self-help group or a major public hospital to see what resources are available to you. Ring your nearest public hospital and ask to speak to the gastroenterology ward to see if the nurse in charge or desk clerk can recommend a support organisation. Not everyone likes to talk about their problems, but it can be good to know that you are not alone by making contact with a group and receiving newsletters or email updates or reading online comments from other members of the group. If you are looking in the telephone directory or searching the Internet for a support group, be wary of profiteers and show caution by preferably selecting a not-for-profit group or organisation that is endorsed or affiliated with the Gastroenterological Society of Australia (GESA).

If you need help with practical things, like housework or having a shower, talk to your doctor or hospital. They may be able to organise for the district nurse in your area to attend to your medical needs. If you need help with household chores, ring your local council, which provides these services, often free of charge or for a small fee, for people in your situation. See the resource section in the back of this book for more contact information.

3
Common complaints

How do you know when you have a gut problem? How can you tell the difference between what are the normal workings of the gastrointestinal tract and what aren't? This chapter aims to clear up some of the common myths and misconceptions about the functions of the GIT. You will find some practical information on things you can do to alleviate basic GIT problems, plus a guide on when you should see your doctor to get further advice.

Before we get started, there are some signs and symptoms that should not be ignored and for which you should see your doctor **immediately**. They are:

- **Severe abdominal pain** that stops you from moving around. It may be associated with sweating, faster pulse and faster breathing than normal or a body temperature above 37.5 degrees Celsius.
- **Diarrhoea and vomiting** that does not stop after 24 hours. With children, a doctor should be seen if it is ongoing after six hours.
- **Vomiting blood.**
- **Bleeding** from your anus or blood in your faeces.

Abdominal pain

Abdominal pain is a common problem experienced by most of us from time to time. It is the body's warning system to tell us that something is not quite right. Sometimes we are able to find a plausible reason for our abdominal pain: we ate too much, pulled a muscle playing tennis, drank too much alcohol, stress at work, or for women it may be at the start of menstruation.

Any pain tends to cause us some anxiety because it hurts or we think that it might be a sign of something more sinister. We all acknowledge pain differently, and what is intense for one person may be described as a mild discomfort by someone else. Fear, stress and anxiety can change our perception of pain. This can make pain difficult to evaluate. But, we do have some skills at doing this. From a young age we learn to recognise different types of pain: dull ache; sharp, stabbing pain; cramping; constant general pain; or a gnawing or burning sensation. These descriptions are useful for helping your doctor work out what is wrong because the site and severity of the pain can be an indication of its cause.

Many episodes of abdominal pain can be resolved by taking an over-the-counter painkiller such as paracetemol. If the pain does not go away by itself and it is affecting your normal day's activities, you need to see a doctor for further advice. A medical practitioner should promptly investigate any pain that gets worse over several hours. If not, you should see someone else.

What is abdominal pain?

Pain is the end result of a message to our brain from the nervous system. The nervous system is a highly complex network of nerves, a bit like a metropolitan road system. The freeways and highways are the major nerve pathways or fibres that travel along the spinal cord to the brain; the minor roads are the smaller nerves that travel down to our peripheries, to our arms and legs.

The streets and cul-de-sacs are the tiny nerve cells, also called pain receptors, which detect a stimulus or source of pain and they transport that message back to the major nerve centres (brain and spinal cord).

When we experience abdominal pain, the nerve cells in the abdomen pick up on a stimulus that is interpreted as being bad for our bodies and a message of 'pain' is sent back up the nerve pathways to the brain. Taking painkillers interferes with the message system so that we don't receive the pain signals for the time that the drug is in our system. Most painkillers do not treat the underlying problem, only the pain. This is why it is important to see a doctor if pain persists once the drug has worn off.

The type of pain we feel changes depending on what the cause is and where it is coming from. In the abdomen, the three major types of pain are **visceral**, **parietal**, and **referred**.

Visceral pain refers to pain messages from the abdominal organs such as the intestines, stomach, liver, and spleen. These organs have few pain receptors compared to other parts of the body and because of this, the pain from these organs is often felt as a dull ache, which is difficult to pinpoint. Sometimes we may not know that we have a problem until the cause leads to stretching or interfering with the membrane that holds and keeps all our abdominal organs in the abdominal cavity, called the **peritoneum**.

The peritoneum has two thin layers: an inside layer (visceral) and outside layer (parietal). The outer layer has many more nerve fibres than the inside layer and abdominal organs. When the outside layer becomes inflamed for some reason, the nerve fibres send a message via the spinal cord to the brain. This is **parietal pain**. It is usually a constant and fairly intense pain, and can be pinpointed to the exact site of the organ.

Referred pain is, as the name suggests, pain that is experienced at a distance from its cause. This is because many pain nerves share the same highways and it can be difficult for the body to tell where the message of pain is coming from. In the gastrointestinal system, a typical type of referred pain is shoulder-tip pain. This is because parts of the peritoneum, particularly those closest to the diaphragm, share the same nerve pathway as the skin over the tip of the shoulder.

One of the problems doctors face when trying to diagnose abdominal pain is that it can be vague because of the limited number of nerve pathways in the abdomen and the sharing of these pathways. Sometimes the abdominal pain may not be caused by a problem in the GIT, but by nearby organs such as the kidneys, bladder, uterus, ovaries, fallopian tubes, gall bladder, pancreas and liver. This is why it is important to get any unresolved pain investigated by a doctor.

What is the difference between acute and chronic pain?

Acute pain is defined as any episode that persists for up to three months. Chronic pain lasts beyond this time.

What causes acute abdominal pain?

The four main causes of abdominal pain are: inflammation; obstruction; too little blood flow to a part of the GIT (ischaemia); and tension (stretching) within a solid organ. The reasons behind these four causes are too numerous to list here. The important point is that any abdominal pain that is stopping you from doing your normal day's activities, or that does not go away after pain relief has worn off, needs to be investigated by your doctor.

What causes chronic abdominal pain?

Chronic abdominal pain can be caused by many physical and psychological causes. It should be investigated by a doctor. The most common cause of chronic abdominal pain is irritable bowel syndrome (IBS).

What are the symptoms of acute abdominal pain?

This depends on the cause of the pain and its location. Pain can be constant or crampy. It can be generalised or specific to one area of the abdomen. The type of pain experienced depends on which of the four causes is responsible.

Inflammation

Organ pain (visceral pain) caused by inflammation that has not affected the peritoneum is more difficult to pinpoint. It is a vague abdominal discomfort.

When inflammation spreads and affects the parietal peritoneum, you can usually pinpoint the pain with a finger. This is because the peritoneum has more nerve endings than an organ, so it is easier to locate the inflammation. This type of pain is usually constant and gets worse with movement and sudden actions such as coughing. It feels momentarily better when you remain still.

Referred pain can occur when the inflammation irritates the outside layer of the peritoneum. This layer has chemical receptors to detect fluids that should not be there, such as blood or gastric secretions that have leaked out because of a perforation or haemorrhage of any part of the GIT. The typical symptoms of referred pain in this instance are shoulder-tip pain, and stiffening of the abdominal muscles called guarding.

Obstruction

If the pain is caused by an obstruction to the bowel, it is usually crampy or colicky, often caused by the body increasing peristalsis in a bid to remove the blockage. It is often severe and comes in waves.

Ischaemia

When parts of the body do not get enough blood, it can cause the tissue to die because of a lack of oxygen to the cells. Pain caused by lack of arterial blood flow is usually of sudden onset, severe and continuous. If it is caused by a blockage to the veins, the pain may develop less suddenly, but it will develop along similar lines.

Organ tension

Swelling of solid organs like the liver causes a pain that is dull and constant. Many things, including bleeding, a clot or a tumour, can cause the swelling. The pain gets worse as the swelling gets worse.

Table 3.1 Site and type of acute abdominal pain

Organ	What it feels like	Where it is felt
Stomach	Constant	Upper abdomen in the middle (epigastric)
Duodenum	Constant	Upper abdomen in the middle (epigastric)
Small intestine	Crampy	Central, near the belly button, or right side
Large intestine	Crampy/Constant	Lower abdomen
Sigmoid colon	Crampy/Constant	Left side of lower abdomen
Gall bladder	Constant	Right side of upper abdomen
Liver	Constant	Right side of upper abdomen
Pancreas	Constant	Upper abdomen in the middle (epigastric)
Ovary/fallopian	Constant	Either side

How to manage acute abdominal pain?

As a general rule, acute abdominal pain should be investigated by a doctor, particularly if the pain is stopping you from going about your daily business and you do not know the cause; your body is trying to tell you something and you need to listen.

What will the doctor do?

A skilled physician will examine you and ask questions about other features of your pain, such as its pattern, frequency, duration and intensity, to help locate the problem. They will observe other general health signs, such as blood pressure, pulse, breathing rate, body temperature and mental alertness, to help work out what is wrong. They may want to ask you questions about your past medical history, family history, medications, recent illnesses, diet, bowel and menstrual habits. You should volunteer any information that you think may be useful. Your doctor may order blood, urinary or faecal tests and abdominal scans to get more information. Depending on the cause of the pain, that is haemorrhage, ischaemia or obstruction, you may need to be hospitalised.

Rectal bleeding

Bleeding from the back passage is rectal bleeding and it is a very common symptom, which almost everyone experiences in their lifetime.

What causes it?

Anything more than spotting should be investigated promptly by your doctor. The vast majority of rectal bleeding is caused by haemorrhoids and is usually of small quantities that cause no more than spotting on the toilet paper and is not serious. Rarely, rectal bleeding can be caused by gastroenteritis, inflammatory bowel disease or diverticular disease, and sometimes it can be caused by polyps or cancer.

When to see the doctor

If the bleeding doesn't settle down in a day or two, or large amounts of blood are passed, enough to be obvious in the toilet bowl, then you should see your doctor. Colonoscopy is often recommended if you are older than 50, have a family history of bowel cancer, or experience lots of bleeding or ongoing bleeding.

How to treat it

When haemorrhoids are the cause, treating any underlying constipation is usually the best first step, as this is the usual cause of the haemorrhoids. Troublesome haemorrhoids can also be treated surgically with a range of treatments, from banding (putting rubber bands over them) to operations to remove them. Treating the underlying constipation is best because haemorrhoids will always eventually return if constipation continues. Treatment of other causes of bleeding needs to be considered with advice from your doctor, and are discussed under the relevant chapter headings in this book.

Bloating

Bloating is a word some people use to describe the feeling of fullness believed to be from having excessive gas in their digestive system.

What causes it?

Eating certain foods and drinking fizzy drinks can cause excessive gas. It can also be caused by swallowing air (see burping below) or it can be a by-product of the normal bacterial breakdown of food in the intestines. Suddenly increasing the amount of fibre in your diet can also increase digestive activity and thereby increase gas production; as can a food intolerance such as wheat if you have coeliac disease. If you have recently suffered a stomach infection such as gastroenteritis, your bacteria levels may have been upset and this can also increase gas production and cause temporary lactose intolerance.

Eating a fatty meal can give the sensation of fullness because the fats slow down the emptying time of the stomach and stay in the stomach for longer. Some women report feeling more bloated just before their period is due; this may be because of hormonal changes causing fluid retention. The contraceptive pill may have a similar effect in some women. Eating salty foods can also cause fluid retention that could be mistaken for bloating.

X-ray studies have shown that people with IBS who complain of bloating often have normal levels of gas in their intestines. This is not to say that they are imagining the problem, but it seems they are more sensitive to the internal actions of their intestines than others and feel discomfort more readily.

How to treat it

Some people find relief from using prebiotic foods and drinks to increase the amount of 'good' bacteria in their gut, which can reduce the amount of gas produced by other gut bacteria. However, more research needs to be done in this area.

What to avoid

Avoid foods that are known to increase gas production when they are broken down in the gut. These include legumes such as lentils, chickpeas and baked beans and vegetables such as Brussels sprouts, cabbage, onions, broccoli and cauliflower. Different foods affect people's digestive systems differently. Foods that can upset some people may not affect you. Some of the possible foods that might be causing the bloating are: asparagus, corn, foods containing a fruit sugar called fructose, foods containing lactose, potatoes, an artificial sweetener called sorbitol, and wheat. It may be worthwhile keeping a diary to record the foods you eat, and work out which ones make you feel bloated. Avoid these foods for a few weeks, and then reintroduce them to your diet one by one to see if they are still troublesome. You should consider talking to a dietitian for their advice. They may want to test you for food intolerances such as fructose malabsorption (see chapter four).

Burping

Burping or belching is the sound of swallowed air escaping from our stomachs via our mouths. The sound the air makes can be just a little squeak or a loud, sometimes guttural noise as the air is pushed out under pressure from a contraction of the abdominal muscles. Belching tends to describe louder burps, but the two terms can be used interchangeably.

What causes it?

We swallow air all the time but we usually don't notice it. When we eat, we also swallow air. If we get excited, we can gulp air. Fizzy drinks contain gas that can make burping or belching worse. Some foods, such as sponge cake, also contain more air than others.

Some people suffer a condition called **aerophagia**, which is the unconscious habit of swallowing air. They can belch regularly with little control. Chewing gum, fizzy drinks and smoking can make the problem worse and these things should be avoided.

When to see the doctor

There is no evidence that burping or belching is harmful. Studies have shown that people who belch excessively usually have no underlying physical problem, and it is most likely occurring out of habit. Some researchers have suggested there may be a link between people who belch regularly and the presence of a hiatus hernia or reflux disease, but this has not been established. Talk to your doctor if you are worried.

How to treat it

Avoid foods and drinks that contain gas. Stop smoking and chewing gum if you have acquired these habits. Some people with aerophagia have had some success at controlling their belching by learning relaxation techniques. Yoga and other meditative therapies may also help.

Constipation

This is something we all experience at some time. Constipation is a symptom, not an illness in its own right. The medical definition for constipation is having a bowel movement fewer than three times a week. However, we are all different and so are our bowels. For some people this can be normal, as can having a bowel action three times a day. Constipation really means that a person is having difficulty ridding the body of faecal waste and they may need to strain to achieve a bowel action. Their faeces may be hard or look like rabbit droppings. Constipation can cause lower abdominal pain, which can be severe.

What causes it?

The reasons we get constipated are many and varied, ranging from something as simple as not drinking enough water to lack of physical activity or not eating enough fibre. Rarely, constipation can be a symptom of serious disease, such as a bowel tumour that is blocking the passage of faeces. Some drugs can cause constipation: examples include codeine and narcotic painkillers, antacids that contain aluminium and calcium, some blood pressure medications, drugs to treat Parkinson's disease, antidepressants, iron tablets, diuretics (drugs that make you wee), and anticonvulsants. Long-term laxative abuse can also cause constipation.

Changes to your routine or lifestyle can cause constipation. Pregnancy is one example, particularly in the third trimester when the mother-to-be may be a little dehydrated and the hormones and pressure of the growing foetus are affecting the bowel's movements. Ageing also changes bowel habits because our metabolism slows and our bowels can get sluggish. Travel can upset our bowels, too. This may be because we forget to drink enough fluids or we do less physical activity. Constipation is a feature of many diseases, including disease of the nervous system, metabolic illnesses such as diabetes, and systemic illnesses such as lupus. Constipation is a problem attributed to many of the gastrointestinal diseases and disorders of the colon and rectum discussed in this book.

Your doctor should investigate ongoing constipation. In some cases, constipation can result from psychological factors that cause us to ignore urges to go to the toilet, such as a phobia of using public toilets.

How to treat it

Remember, constipation is a symptom, so treat the underlying cause if you know what it is. If you don't know, see your doctor. Ongoing constipation can be the symptom of something more serious and it should not be ignored—you need to see your doctor. Likewise, if constipation is a chronic problem, you need to seek medical advice.

Listed below are the changes you can make to your diet and lifestyle that can make a big difference to constipation and stop it recurring.

Diet
- **Increase your fluid intake**—Aim for about 2 litres a day, preferably water.
- **Increase fibre**—Aim to eat 25 to 30 grams of fibre a day. This can be made easier by increasing your intake of fruit and vegetables. See chapters four and nine for more information.
- **Eat regularly**—Get your body in a routine. Try to eat meals of similar sizes well spaced throughout the day so that your body has time to digest and absorb nutrients before the next meal.

Lifestyle changes

- **Increase your level of exercise**—Find an activity you enjoy and do it a few times a week for at least 30 minutes. Try and build it into your day; this makes it easier to continue for the long term. Walk the dog or get off the train or bus one stop early and walk home.
- **Establish a routine where possible**—Your body will thank you for it. Try and eat regularly. Don't ignore urges to go to the toilet as this can make constipation worse; if you do this, think about the reasons why. If it is because you dislike public toilets, find a place you can tolerate such as a favourite coffee shop, library or gymnasium. If you don't like going at work, try the toilets on another floor.

What to avoid

- **Tea, coffee or any drink high in caffeine such as some energy drinks, and alcohol**—These can be dehydrating, making constipation worse.
- **Reliance on laxatives**—Long-term use can weaken the muscle tone of the bowel causing a reverse effect from the one intended, making constipation worse.
- **Certain foods**—These will vary from person to person. Some people find foods with little or no fibre are a big problem. These include cheese, ice cream and some processed foods. To better understand which foods affect your bowels, keep a food diary for a few weeks and make a note of when you get constipated. Try eliminating these foods for a while to see if it helps. Gradually reintroduce them one by one. If the constipation gets worse, exclude that food from your diet.
- **Drugs that make constipation worse**—While it may not always be possible to stop taking these, you should talk to your doctor about your medication options.

- **Inactivity**—Increase your physical activity. This can be great for getting the bowels moving.
- **Ignoring urges**—This can make constipation worse.

Diarrhoea

Diarrhoea (spelt diarrhea in the United States) is another symptom that we all experience from time to time. It is often described as a 'loose' bowel action. It means that our faeces is not in its normal solid state, and is liquid or watery instead. We may also experience urgency, and may need to go the toilet several times a day. Diarrhoea can be acute (short-term) or chronic (more than three months). Depending on the cause, diarrhoea can be preceded by crampy abdominal pain (colic). While diarrhoea is a very common symptom, it can be a very serious problem if ignored or not treated. In third-world countries, diarrhoea, usually resulting from infections such as cholera, dysentery and botulism, is the leading cause of infant deaths, killing more than 1.5 million children a year.

What causes it?

Many things can cause diarrhoea, including: infection by a virus, bacterium, fungus or parasite; food poisoning; food allergies or intolerances such as lactose intolerance and coeliac disease; excesses of certain chemicals such as magnesium; anxiety; too much alcohol; changes to the diet; drugs, particularly antibiotics; damage to the intestines or their blood supply; cancer, hormone and nervous system problems; and GIT diseases, including many of the illnesses discussed in the following chapters. Diarrhoea can also be caused by constipation. This is called **spurious diarrhoea** and it happens when the faecal material caught behind the hard faeces that is clogging the bowel and causing constipation seeps past the blockage giving the appearance of diarrhoea. Once properly diagnosed by your doctor, this should be treated as outlined under the heading constipation.

Diarrhoea often results when fluid is not reabsorbed in the large bowel, which is a normal process of the gastrointestinal system. There are a few reasons for this:

- Too much fluid moves from the body into the bowel and it is not reabsorbed in the large bowel. This occurs with gastro-enteritis and travellers' diarrhoea.
- The nervous system and hormones, which control the speed of the movement of the bowel (peristalsis), are sped up and the fluid does not have a chance to be reabsorbed back into the body. This can happen when we are anxious, the bowel is irritated as in IBS, or there is an underlying hormonal or nervous system problem, such as long-standing diabetes.
- The concentration of salt and other chemicals is altered, or too much liquid is drunk. Both of these factors can influence the movement of fluid in the body and the reabsorption of water in the bowel. This can happen with certain medications or foods, such as sugar-free chewing gum.

When to see the doctor

If the diarrhoea is chronic, see your doctor as it needs to be investigated. If it is acute and does not settle down after a day or so, also consult your doctor. See a doctor sooner if it involves:

- Severe dehydration
- A very young child (under two years) or elderly person (they get dehydrated much more quickly)
- Blood in the stool or toilet bowl
- High body temperature (above 38°C) with signs of a fever, sweating or shaking.

Your doctor will ask questions about medications, diet and bowel habits. They will want to feel your abdomen and may need to examine the rectum using a gloved finger. They might organise a blood test and stool sample to see if you have an infection. Other tests that might be needed depending on your symptoms include an X-ray of the abdomen and colonoscopy. Depending on the cause, your doctor may prescribe antibiotics. If dehydration is severe, you may need to be hospitalised and have a drip inserted to restore fluid.

How to treat it

When gastroenteritis, alcohol, food poisoning or dietary changes are the cause, then the diarrhoea is likely to be short-lived. The important thing is to keep up your fluids so that you do not become dehydrated. Use rehydration preparations from your pharmacist if you have had muscle aches and pains from the effects of dehydration.

Wash your hands before touching things in case the diarrhoea is infectious. Always wash your hands with soap after each toilet visit. For the same reason, do not be involved in food preparation or feeding others until the diarrhoea has resolved. If the diarrhoea is caused by an infection, take some time off work so that you don't pass it on to others—it is highly contagious through touch.

If you have changed your diet to a high-fibre diet, go back to your previous diet and introduce fibre more gradually over a month or so. Be careful about taking antidiarrhoeal medication unless you know what the cause is and have discussed it with your pharmacist or doctor. These medications usually work by slowing down peristalsis and can be dangerous if used incorrectly. They should NOT be used in children or elderly people unless directed by your doctor.

What to avoid

- Suspected contaminated food that may have caused the diarrhoea.
- Fluids that are dehydrating such as alcohol, tea and coffee.
- Eating too much—Your intestines will need a rest from food for a day or so. Start off by eating easy-to-digest foods such as toast without butter, dry biscuits, plain white rice and soup.
- High fibre foods, milk and milk products (yoghurt and probiotic yoghurt is okay though) until your bowel has fully recovered after a few weeks.

Flatulence (wind)

Perhaps better known as farting or 'passing wind', flatulence is the movement of gas out of the body from the anus. The gas is sometimes referred to as flatus and usually contains a mix of gases including hydrogen and methane.

What causes it?

Like burping, it is caused by gas in the digestive system that comes from the mechanical and chemical breakdown of food. The difference is that the gas is trapped in the lower GIT and the quickest exit is the rear end. One study of healthy students found the average person did about thirteen farts a day. There is no truth to the adage that ladies do not pass wind—it is more likely that they are just more discreet about its passage by removing themselves from social company. Flatulence can be noisy, depending on the force of the expulsion of gas from the anal sphincter; although, because the sphincter is under our conscious influence, we can exert some control over the timing of its release. Flatus can smell because of its methane component. The odour also depends on the variety of micro-organisms in the bowel that are responsible for some of the chemical digestion of food matter.

Is it harmful?

Usually not; however, because methane and hydrogen are combustible gases, any bowel procedures that may involve a heat source, such as electrocautery used to burn polyps, should not be done unless the patient has had a proper bowel preparation to minimise gas production.

How to treat it

Diet is the best way to treat excess gas. The breakdown of some foods produces more gas than others. Avoid foods that are known for their gas production such as baked beans and other legumes, as well as some vegetables including onions and vegetables from the *Brassica* family like Brussels sprouts and cabbage (see chapter four). Carbohydrate foods produce little gas because these are usually fully absorbed in the small intestine. Studies have found that drugs that claim to prevent flatus are of little benefit.

Floating stools

These are bowel actions that float. Healthy people can have floating stools. It doesn't necessarily mean there is a problem.

What causes it?

It was once thought that they were always caused by high fat content in the stool. Often, it is only a result of having a higher content of gas in the stool than normal, or malabsorption of nutrients. These two factors can be caused by dietary changes or a recent infection causing diarrhoea. Curiously, some medical conditions such as cystic fibrosis, coeliac disease, short bowel syndrome or an enzyme deficiency have been blamed for producing floating stools.

How to treat it

First, work out if it is a problem that needs to be treated. If there are no other symptoms, you need not worry. If it is a problem related to other symptoms, see your doctor to treat the underlying cause. If you have recently had gastroenteritis, your stools will return to normal when you recover from the illness.

Gastroenteritis

The term gastroenteritis usually refers to an acute infection of the bowel.

What causes it?

Gastroenteritis is commonly caused by a virus or occasionally by bacteria, especially associated with reheated chicken, rice and take-away foods. The incubation period for gastroenteritis is generally about twelve hours, meaning that you would start feeling unwell about twelve hours after exposure to the infection. Symptoms generally include diarrhoea, vomiting, nausea and some crampy abdominal pain. Luckily, gastroenteritis almost always resolves after a couple of days. **Food poisoning** is different to gastroenteritis. It is caused by eating stale or rotten food, containing a toxin usually from contamination with bacteria, rather than by catching an infection. The most common source of food poisoning is from eating spoiled seafood. Symptoms can start about an hour after eating the food. It causes more vomiting than gastroenteritis and the food poisoning usually settles down within 24 hours.

How to treat it

The best way to manage gastroenteritis or food poisoning is to have plenty of fluids, and possibly drink rehydration solutions, such as Gastrolyte, in more severe cases. Even when vomiting is frequent, sipping small amounts of water often can be more successful than you may think.

What to avoid

Although it is important to maintain a good fluid intake while unwell, it is probably best to avoid solid foods initially, and rich, fatty foods for a couple of days—these will make diarrhoea worse. Some people can also experience milder symptoms for a few weeks after an infection, commonly attributed to post-infectious IBS. This is probably caused from damage to the bowel lining by an acute infection, and resolves as the bowel lining heals. Sometimes this can also lead to temporary lactose intolerance, so avoid dairy drinks and food products.

Haemorrhoids

There are many myths about haemorrhoids, or piles. Contrary to old wives' tales, they are not caused by sitting on cold surfaces, sitting for too long or lifting heavy objects. Haemorrhoids are a natural occurrence in the body. They are specific parts of the inside of the anal canal where the arteries join veins, called the **anal cushions** (haemorrhoid is another name for 'anal cushion'). They can become a problem when they dilate and/or drop down or **prolapse**. In more extreme cases, they can drop low enough that they can be seen just outside the anus. When the anal cushions prolapse outside the anal canal, the tissue is exposed to harsher conditions than when inside the body and this can cause the tissue to dry out, making it susceptible to more bleeding and itchiness. If a clot forms in the haemorrhoid, it will usually cause pain.

What are the signs and symptoms of haemorrhoids?

Haemorrhoids can be uncomfortable and itchy. Bleeding is the most common sign. More men than women get haemorrhoids. They are usually not very painful, unless a blood clot forms. If there is severe pain in the anal area, your doctor should look for another cause if no clot is found. When they bleed, it is bright red blood. On defecation the blood can drip into the toilet bowl. If the prolapse is severe, the haemorrhoid can bleed for no obvious reason and it may be enough to seep through the clothes. Very occasionally, haemorrhoids can cause minor faecal incontinence.

What causes it?

It is thought that the anal cushions prolapse when there is too much straining during defecation usually because of chronic constipation. Straining weakens the muscles that hold the cushions in place. At first, they may slip down for a few hours before moving back to their correct position. In severe cases, the muscles are so weak that they are unable to keep the cushions in place, and gravity and straining causes the cushions to swell making it impossible for them to return to their correct position.

How to treat it

The key to stopping haemorrhoids forming is to avoid straining when going to the toilet. Simple ways to do this are: go to the toilet as soon as you get the urge; drink lots of water and eat fibre to avoid constipation; and don't read on the toilet, as this can be a distraction that can slow things down and lead to straining.

If the haemorrhoids have prolapsed, they can be injected with a solution or have a rubber band put around them. Both procedures make haemorrhoids smaller and should alleviate the symptoms. If the haemorrhoids are severely prolapsed or other treatment methods have failed, they need to be surgically removed.

Halitosis (bad breath)

Halitosis is unpleasant smelling breath that we may not be aware of but may be noticeable to other people when we breathe out.

What causes it?

Halitosis is common in healthy people. It can occur if we get dehydrated, drink too much coffee, smoke cigarettes, take certain medication, eat particular foods such as onions, garlic, broccoli or leeks, or suffer a dry mouth condition known as **xerostomia** caused by a medical problem or medication side effect. Halitosis is also a common complaint just after waking up from a long sleep when the mouth is dry and bacteria levels in the mouth have increased. Another common cause is bacteria attached to tiny food bits stuck in the teeth or throat.

Occasionally, the cause may be a more serious reason. It is a good idea to see a dentist to make sure there are no mouth or dental problems such as gum disease, a tooth cavity, mouth sores or oral thrush. These conditions tend to increase bacteria levels and therefore halitosis. Halitosis can also be a symptom of respiratory diseases, ranging from the mild, such as sinusitis, a common cold or inflammation of the lung, to the serious, such as a tumour in the respiratory tract, mouth, nose or throat. Liver disease and systemic diseases such as diabetes also cause specific odours. In liver disease, the exhaled breath can take on a musty smell. In diabetes, the exhaled breath can have a fruity odour.

How to treat it

Treatment depends on the cause. If it is a simple problem in a healthy person, then changes to mouth care and diet may be enough to fix it. Good oral hygiene is important. This involves regular brushing and flossing, and periodic visits to the dentist.

Dietary changes can also help. Low-fat diets and increasing your intake of fruit and vegetables can change the acidity in the mouth and increase saliva, which is good for reducing bacteria. If a dry mouth is the problem, you may need to review your medications, as this is the most common cause; drink more water and try measures that increase saliva flow such as sugar-free chewing gum. Gum with sugar can increase bacteria levels and make halitosis worse. If the cause is a fungus, such as oral candidiasis (thrush), antifungal drugs are needed.

If the halitosis is caused by something more serious, the underlying disease needs to be treated by your doctor.

What to avoid

Foods that contain high levels of sulphur, such as leeks, onions, garlic, broccoli and radishes, should be avoided. Also avoid foods that increase the bacteria levels in your mouth, such as sugary foods, chewing gum containing sugar and mouth washes with sugar or alcohol, as these dry the mouth and can make the problem worse.

Hiccups

Hiccups are an involuntary reflex that most healthy people experience from time to time. It is thought that the reflex is triggered when we breathe in and the glottis is closed. When we breathe in and out, the glottis is normally open. The **glottis** is a flap in the throat that closes to stop food going into our lungs when we swallow. The sound and the sensation of the hiccup are caused by the sudden end to our breathing in, despite very strong chest muscle contractions, caused by the glottis closing. Each hiccup lasts about one second.

Very rarely, hiccups may last more than 24 hours. In such cases the condition is called **intractable hiccups** and a more serious underlying cause needs to be investigated immediately.

What causes hiccups?

The trigger for hiccups is not always obvious. It can be triggered by interference with the nerve pathways caused by a very full stomach, emotion, drinking alcohol or sudden changes in temperature.

More serious causes of hiccups can be caused by reflux, small bowel obstruction, blockage in the oesophagus, problems with the nerves of the diaphragm (the very large band of muscle under the lungs), pressure on the diaphragm, problems with the nervous system or brain, or changes to blood chemistry caused by metabolic disorders or drugs.

How to treat them

There are some terrific fables about how to treat hiccups, including: prayers to St Jude, the Patron Saint of Hopeless Causes; placing your fingers in your ears; inhaling from a paper bag; drinking water upside-down (a difficult task); swallowing large-grained sugar; swallowing when you think the next hiccup is due; coughing; sneezing; getting angry; and even having sex. None of these methods has been proved to work, nor disproved for that matter either. They may appear to work because they are a distraction from the problem, which usually goes away by itself after several minutes. Perhaps the easiest and safest treatment is to drink a glass of cold water, which is thought to settle the nerve pathways that caused the hiccups.

Intractable hiccups

When hiccups last for more than 24 hours they are known as intractable hiccups. This is a very disabling condition, often with a serious underlying cause, and needs to be investigated by your doctor immediately. It is usually treated with a drug called chlorpromazine (Largactil).

Itchy bottom

Also called **pruritus ani**, this is a very common condition that can vary from being a mild annoyance to severe itching and pain. Many people with this problem do not seek medical help. A five-year study found it affected about 50 per cent of the general population.

What causes it?

The causes are many, but the exact reason for the itch may never be discovered. Sometimes the skin around the anus may be cracked or chaffed because of dryness. It can also be caused by mild faecal seepage or mucus produced by the rectum that goes unnoticed. This irritates the skin and causes the itchiness. Other causes can include underlying problems such as haemorrhoids, anal tear, warts, skin tags, which are harmless, small folds of excess skin that hang from the body, cancer, fistula, skin infections such as fungi, bacteria or parasites. Threadworms are a common cause of itchy bottom in children, but rarely seen in adults. The problem could also be caused by skin diseases such as eczema and psoriasis, or by very sensitive skin that may be irritated by underwear or topical creams.

What to do about it

Inspect the area with a mirror to see if you can find any obvious problems. If the skin looks dry and cracked, talk to your pharmacist about a low-irritant cream to moisturise the area. Keep the area clean and wear undergarments made of low-irritant materials such as pure cotton. Use soft toilet paper or try alcohol-free baby wipes. If you have recently changed washing powders, stop using the new brand and see if that helps. Scratching the itch will make it worse, so try to resist. If it doesn't resolve after a few days, see your doctor.

Mucus

Mucus is a slimy, clear, white or yellow secretion with the consistency of jelly. Mucus is produced by many parts of the body to protect it from harsh internal conditions.

What causes it?

In the gastrointestinal system, mucus is made throughout the GIT and its purpose is to protect the inner lining of the stomach and intestines from the strong digestive enzymes and acids that work to break down food. Mucus also lubricates the partially digested food matter so that it can move through the system, as well as the unwanted matter so that it can be excreted as waste in the form of faeces.

What to do about it

Most times we are unaware of the mucus made in our GIT because the intestines reabsorb it or it is mixed up in the faeces and excreted. Occasionally, if we have been unwell, the faeces may not be properly formed and we may notice it, or we may produce more mucus because the intestinal wall where it is made has become inflamed or infected. Mucus is a symptom of this inflammation process which is caused by several bowel diseases including IBS, IBD, bacterial infection or bowel obstruction. Also, people who have had bowel surgery and no longer use their rectum to store bowel actions, because they have had it detached from their large bowel, sometimes notice mucus leaving the anus. This happens because the mucous membrane of the rectum still continues to make the mucus. If it is a new symptom or you are worried about it, see your doctor.

Nausea

Nausea is the sensation of feeling like you are going to vomit; however, it may or may not be followed with vomiting.

What causes it?

The nerve pathways involved in feeling the sensation of nausea are quite complex. Nausea can be caused by a problem in the stomach, such as an ulcer, or alternatively it can be caused by diseases affecting the hypothalamus, an area of the brain responsible for nausea, or occasionally psychological factors such as stressful situations. Diseases affecting the hypothalamus are rare but can include brain tumours, or conditions outside the brain that release chemicals that act on the hypothalamus, such as certain types of cancer, and less sinister causes such as being pregnant.

What to do about it

Persistent nausea can be potentially serious as well as very disabling, and is usually best sorted out by consulting your doctor. There are medications that can be prescribed to ease the symptoms. Tests that can be helpful for identifying the underlying problem include blood tests and endoscopy. In the rare occurrence that a brain tumor is suspected, a scan of the head may be required.

Vomiting

The medical word for vomiting is **emesis**—it is one of the body's reflexes causing the forceful projection of food or liquid out of the stomach or small intestine back up into the gullet (oesophagus) and out of the mouth.

What causes it?

Most of us have experienced vomiting at some stage. It is the body's natural mechanism for ridding the GIT of unwanted substances. These substances can be infected foods, too much alcohol, drugs or medications, or an infection from a virus, bacterium, fungus or parasite. Sometimes we vomit because the nervous pathways, receptors or hormones that transfer messages to the parts of the brain involved in the vomiting reflex are interfered with by something such as extreme pain, a disease, tumour, or changes to the chemistry in our blood caused by a metabolic illness, kidney failure or post surgery.

It may be triggered by something less serious, such as hormonal upsets as is the case in a minority of pregnancies; or perhaps something that has upset the vomiting receptors in the brain, such as constant movement experienced in seasickness, or an awful smell or sight, or extreme emotions—this is why people in movies who stumble on a murder scene often vomit. Another reflex can be triggered if we are in danger of choking, which also leads to vomiting. This is called the **gag reflex**. Vomiting may be self-induced by physically activating the gag reflex as is the case with psychiatric conditions such as eating disorders.

Before we vomit, we often get warning signs. These include nausea and increased salivation in the mouth called **waterbrash**, which occurs in anticipation of vomiting and is designed to protect the enamel of the teeth from the stomach acids when the contents are expelled. Other bodily changes that occur during vomiting include the reversal of peristalsis, called **retroperistalsis**, which moves the stomach contents back up the oesophagus. This is helped by contractions of the abdominal muscles, relaxation of the lower oesophageal sphincter, and the closure of the glottis to protect the lungs from the vomited contents going into them.

When to see the doctor

You should see your doctor **immediately** if:

- A poison has been ingested or is suspected as the cause of the vomiting.
- You are vomiting large amounts of blood, matter that looks like coffee grounds, or faeces.
- You are vomiting continuously.
- You develop a stiff neck or headache, or your eyes become very sensitive to light.
- There are signs of severe dehydration, including: not needing to urinate or producing small amounts of dark brown urine; unable to produce tears; very dry mouth; top of head appears

sunken in babies; skin loses its elasticity and stays wrinkled if pinched; and feeling tired and unable to concentrate.

Remember that children and elderly people feel the effects of dehydration more quickly and you should not hesitate to take them to seek medical advice.

In all cases, if medical help is required, your doctor may need to insert a drip to get body fluid levels back to normal. A drug to stop the vomiting, called an **anti-emetic**, may be given through the drip. Your doctor will ask questions about diet, recent travel, bowel habits, medications and other symptoms you might have experienced. They may do a series of tests including blood tests, and, once the vomiting has calmed down, order a stomach X-ray and endoscopy.

How to treat it

If the vomiting is not severe and is not causing any of the problems outlined above, the important thing is to keep up your fluids. Drink sips of water, about 30 ml every 10 minutes or so. Check the amount and colour of your urine to make sure you are not becoming too dehydrated. Avoid eating until the vomiting has stopped for several hours. When you do feel hungry and want to eat, start slowly with toast (no butter), and dry biscuits and soup for the first day or so, to give your stomach and intestines a rest.

Further information

Medical contacts

Gastroenterological Society of Australia (GESA)
145 Macquarie Street

Sydney NSW 2000
Phone: (02) 9256 5454
Fax: (02) 9241 4586
Email: gesa@gesa.org.au
Website: www.gesa.org.au

British Society of Gastroenterology
3 St Andrews Place
Regents Park
London NW1 4LB
Phone: +44 (0) 20 7935 3150
Fax: +44 (0) 20 7487 3734
Email: bsg@mailbox.ulcc.ac.uk
Website: www.bsg.org.uk

American Gastroenterological Association (AGA)
National Office
4930 Del Ray Avenue
Bethesda, MD 20814
Phone: +1 (301) 654 2055
Fax: +1 (301) 654 5920
Email: member@gastro.org
Website: www.gastro.org

Useful websites

The Australian Broadcasting Corporation has a health site with useful information and web links about the GIT and other bowel disorders: www.abc.net.au/health/default.htm.

An online information service called GastroNet set up by Australian gastroenterologists and health professionals includes dietary information for IBS and other digestive disorders: www.gastro.net.au.

A useful Victorian government health website that has information on different gastrointestinal complaints can be found at: www.betterhealth.vic.gov.au.

The Digestive Disorders Foundation is the British charity that operates under the name CORE. CORE is the UK's Digestive Disorders foundation's health website on GIT problems containing information on many diseases and symptoms: www.corecharity.org.uk.

The National Digestive Diseases Information Clearinghouse (NDDIC) is a US government health information service. The website is easy to follow with excellent explanations of GIT symptoms and common complaints: www.digestive.niddk. nih.gov.

4
Irritable bowel syndrome (IBS)

I remember having abdominal pain when I was at school but my mum never took me to see a doctor. I felt bloated all the time. A friend told me to have less dairy in my diet because when I ate dairy foods I got diarrhoea. But it is not just dairy that brings it on. When we went away to Bali last year, I had diarrhoea for six weeks. The pain and bloating was getting worse, to the point where I didn't feel like going out for lunch with my friends in case it came on. When I finally saw my local doctor, he told me there was nothing wrong and suggested it was probably caused by anxiety. Still, he referred me to a gastroenterologist who did a blood test for coeliac disease, which was negative. The gastro-enterologist said I probably had irritable bowel syndrome. He told me to make some changes to my diet, to stop working so much overtime, and to take some tablets to relax the bowel. It has made a difference. I still get bloated sometimes, particularly when I'm stressed. I guess when I think about it I have had IBS most of my life. At least I can put a name to it now.

Alice, 28, architect and mother of two

What is irritable bowel syndrome (IBS)?

IBS can be a painful, chronic condition that usually presents with abdominal pain and altered bowel habit—diarrhoea, constipation, or alternating episodes of both. It is usually a condition that waxes and wanes.

It is often difficult to diagnose because there is no single test to confirm the condition, and it has many of the symptoms of other gut disorders.

People with IBS may experience some or all of these problems:

- Cramping abdominal pain, often in the morning
- Feeling bloated
- Abdominal distension, often after meals or commonly occurs at night
- Passing wind
- Changed bowel habits, such as going to the toilet more than three times a day, or going less than three times a week
- Pain that may be relieved by opening bowels
- Toilet troubles, such as straining, urgency or a feeling of incomplete defecation
- Passing mucus
- Funny-shaped stools, descriptions include anything from stools like rabbit droppings to toothpaste.

Doctors call it a functional condition because the bowel does not appear to be physically damaged when it is examined. Instead, it is the function of the bowel that seems to be affected by IBS. In past years IBS has also been referred to as 'colitis', 'mucous colitis', 'spastic colon' and 'spastic bowel'. None of these terms is an accurate description of the condition and they have therefore been replaced by irritable bowel syndrome.

IBS sufferers may also experience other functional gut symptoms such as:

- Heartburn
- Dyspepsia, an ulcer-type pain
- Globus sensation, the feeling of something stuck in your throat
- Nausea
- Excessive belching.

Those with IBS may also have some non-gut symptoms such as:

- Tiredness
- Painful periods in women
- Pain during sex
- Headache
- Problems sleeping
- Sensitive bladder
- Fibromyalgia, which is aches and pains in the joints and muscles.

Medical professionals classify IBS into three categories. They are:

- **IBS with diarrhoea-predominance (IBS-D)**—This is associated with abdominal pain or discomfort and frequent, urgent bowel movements (more than three per day) with loose watery stools; there may also be a feeling of incomplete emptying after a bowel movement.
- **IBS with constipation-predominance (IBS-C)**—This is associated with abdominal pain or discomfort, fewer than three bowel movements per week, hard lumpy stools, and straining during bowel movements; there may also be a feeling of fullness or bloating.
- **Alternating IBS (IBS-A)**—This is associated with abdominal pain or discomfort and alternating constipation and diarrhoea.

There may be symptom overlap between these different types of IBS.

Who does IBS affect?

IBS is very common and affects about one in five Australians. Women are twice as likely as men to be affected—although this figure may be skewed because women are more likely to go to a doctor than men. Many people affected by IBS do not seek medical help, so the problem is likely to be bigger than estimated. That said, IBS is one of the main reasons why people visit their doctor. It is the cause of many sick days from work, and is very costly to the community in terms of medical appointments, hospital visits and drugs.

People with busy, demanding lifestyles and fast-paced, stressful jobs are more at risk of suffering IBS than others. We have all heard of 'nerves in our tummy' when we have to perform. This is a basic example of the complex relationship between stress and its effects on our bowels. We all feel stress at times during our lives, perhaps it is when we apply for a home loan, sit an exam or go for a job interview, but some people seem to encounter these symptoms more than others. For example, doctors are reporting, anecdotally, an increase in the number of students from second-generation Australian families with IBS. One theory is that children of immigrants are stressed because they feel pressure, either real or perceived, to perform well at school and in their careers, to please their parents. IBS is a rare condition in developing countries such as Africa, which also suggests that a stressful, busy lifestyle is an important factor in causing the disease.

What causes IBS?

No one really knows. Doctors believe IBS is caused by a number of things that together can trigger the disease.

It is known that some people with IBS may be more aware of the inside workings of their stomach and gut, which are normally not consciously registered by other people. This awareness can be felt as pain. The term used to describe this experience is **visceral hypersensitivity**.

Other sufferers are believed to have a small or large bowel that does not contract properly when food passes through the digestive system. There seems to be a problem with the coordination of the muscle contractions in the bowel. This is called **disordered motility**.

Diet also plays a role in IBS. It is thought that some people may be intolerant to particular short-chain carbohydrates (sugars), which are not properly absorbed in the small intestine and pass into the large intestine where they are fermented by bacteria. This process produces excessive gas, which leads to pain, bloating and wind. This theory is being rigorously researched and is discussed later in this chapter.

About 25 per cent of people with IBS begin to get symptoms after experiencing a stomach or bowel infection, otherwise known as **gastroenteritis**.

As mentioned earlier, stress is also thought to trigger the disease, as is mental illness. Some studies have found a link between sexual or physical abuse in the past or present and IBS. There is evidence that stressful life events increase the risk of IBS. People already suffering anxiety or depression may feel IBS symptoms more intensely when under duress. Doctors have noticed a trend that suggests people with certain personality traits, such as a Type A personality—often high achievers who have a lot of pressure and stress in their lives—are vulnerable to experiencing IBS.

Other sufferers may have a relative with IBS. Research has found that having a relative with IBS does slightly increase the risk of other family members experiencing IBS—but a word of caution, the increased risk is very small.

Some doctors believe that the loops of the large bowel hang lower in people with IBS, which in turn affects the bowel's ability to contract properly. This is called **redundant colon**. This theory has yet to be scientifically proven and divides the medical community; some doctors dismiss it as a factor that causes the disease.

How do you know you have IBS?

It is unlikely that you will be told you have IBS straightaway. IBS sufferers have many of the symptoms that could be attributed to other conditions. Your doctor needs to be sure that you don't have something else that may appear to be IBS. See Table 4.1 for a list of some of the problems that can look like IBS. As IBS is a condition that comes and goes, your doctor will want to know the history of when you first started getting symptoms. It is useful to keep a diary or mark the date on the calendar when you get symptoms. This will make charting your history much easier.

IBS usually follows a pattern and based on this, and the results of the tests outlined below, your doctor can make a diagnosis. People with IBS often present with symptoms that come and go for a total of twelve or more weeks (usually non-consecutive weeks) a year. However, this medical criterion is now considered too narrow by many health professionals and it is possible to have IBS without fitting this rule.

How is IBS diagnosed?

The first things your doctor will do are listen to you and take notes. This is called **taking a history**. They will want to know what physical problems you have experienced: Is there pain? Where is it? How often do you go to the toilet? What happens when you go to the toilet? How many days or weeks do these symptoms go on for?

They may also want to physically examine you. This normally includes things like taking your blood pressure, pressing on your abdomen and possibly even carrying out a rectal examination to check for abnormalities.

Once your doctor has taken your history and performed a physical examination then, depending on your individual experience, they will order some tests. Typically, the tests include those listed below:

Blood tests

A sample of your blood will be taken, usually from your arm. This blood will be sent to the laboratory to check things such as iron, haemoglobin and other blood components. Depending on your symptoms, your doctor may ask the lab to check your hormone levels from your thyroid gland and your calcium levels; and they may also do a blood test to rule out coeliac disease.

A stool sample

You may be asked to provide a sample of your stool to be sent to the laboratory to see if you have an infection.

A colonoscopy (with or without a biopsy)

If you are experiencing IBS symptoms for the first time, you may need a colonoscopy, particularly if you have noticed blood in your stools or have had unexplained weight loss. A gastroenterologist usually does this. It involves using a colonoscope to look inside the bowel to see if there is any damage. Sometimes biopsies are taken to look more closely at the bowel lining under a microscope. Biopsies are taken with a small instrument that is similar to tweezers. Only very small samples are taken, and it is quite safe. Very little tissue is taken; if it bleeds it is usually a minute amount. Biopsies are painless because there are no nerve endings on the lining of the bowel, though sometimes the colonoscopy procedure can be uncomfortable. It can take between five minutes and 30 minutes, and is usually done under sedation. See chapter two for more information.

Gynaecological examination

Most women with abdominal pain will need a gynaecological examination to rule out a gynaecological cause.

If it is not IBS, then what?

Before you are diagnosed with IBS, it is very important to rule out other illnesses that may have similar symptoms. Also, inflammatory bowel disease (IBD) is a very different problem that should not be confused with IBS. They may sound similar, but the treatment and diseases are quite separate. Do not panic if your doctor is investigating for another cause of your abdominal pain and changed bowel habits. This is an important step before any diagnosis of IBS can be made with confidence. The diagnosis is important because it will determine how you are treated and the effectiveness of the treatment. Some of the conditions that can be confused with IBS, their symptoms and treatment are listed in Table 4.1.

Treating IBS

A number of things can be done to ease the symptoms of IBS. As discussed, the major influences on the disease are diet, medications, lifestyle and emotional factors. Preferably, if changes can be made to your diet and lifestyle, there may be less need for the use of medications. So let's start with diet.

Table 4.1 Conditions that might be considered before diagnosing IBS

Condition	*Symptoms	*Tests
Inflammatory bowel disease (IBD)		
IBD includes ulcerative colitis and Crohn's disease. IBD is a chronic illness with inflammation of the bowel. See chapter eight for detailed information.	Abdominal pain Diarrhoea Blood and mucus in stools Weight loss Tiredness Anaemia Skin and eye problems Wind Bloating	Colonoscopy Barium X-ray Blood tests
Coeliac disease		
An intolerance to gluten, a protein found in wheat, barley, rye and oats. Associated with other diseases like Type 1 diabetes. See chapter seven for more detailed information.	Abdominal pain Wind Bloating Diarrhoea and constipation Weight loss Malnutrition Osteoporosis	Blood test Endoscopy
Lactose intolerance		
Unable to absorb lactose, which is found in milk and some dairy products such as soft cheese. Particularly common in people of Asian descent. Caused by a congenital lack of an enzyme, called lactase, that breaks down lactose.	Diarrhoea Wind Abdominal pain Bloating	Breath test Dietary trial

Table 4.1 Conditions that might be considered before diagnosing IBS *continued*

Condition	*Symptoms	*Tests
Medication side effects	Abdominal pain Wind Bloating Diarrhoea or constipation Vomiting and nausea Reflux	Trial of removing or changing medications if possible; Blood test
Cancer of the colon Changes to the cells in the large bowel. Initially there may be few symptoms other than traces of blood in the stool.	Abdominal pain Blood or mucus in stool Weight loss Anorexia (lack of appetite) Tiredness Diarrhoea and/or constipation	Colonoscopy Blood test Stool test for blood CT scan
Diverticulitis Inflammation of pockets in the large bowel. Associated with older age and low-fibre diets. For more detailed information see chapter nine.	Abdominal pain Diarrhoea Fever	Blood tests CT scan Colonoscopy
Pancreatitis Inflammation of a gland, the pancreas, that makes enzymes for digestion and also insulin. Often caused by gall stones or alcohol.	Severe abdominal pain Vomiting Sometimes jaundice (yellow skin)	Blood tests CT scan Ultrasound

Table 4.1 Conditions that might be considered before diagnosing IBS *continued*

Condition	*Symptoms	*Tests
Gall stones Only cause trouble when they are blocked in the gall bladder or bile duct and cause an obstruction.	Episodic abdominal pain Sometimes jaundice (yellow skin)	Blood tests Ultrasound
Giardiasis Caused by a parasite that lives in the gut. The source may be untreated water, unwashed foods, unwashed hands, raw meat and pets. Often treated (without a definite diagnosis) with antibiotics.	Abdominal pain Diarrhoea Wind Vomiting and nausea	Stool sample Treatment with antibiotics Endoscopy
Thyroid disease A problem with the thyroid gland in the throat leading to an oversupply or undersupply of important hormones.	Diarrhoea or constipation Abdominal pain Bloating and wind Tired or overexcited Weight changes	Blood test—thyroid function test
Eating disorders A mental illness leading to intentional food deprivation or sporadic consumption of food followed by induced vomiting. The two most common eating disorders are anorexia nervosa and bulimia.	Vomiting Anorexia (lack of appetite) Diarrhoea Constipation Weight fluctuations Tiredness	Psychiatric assessment Blood tests

Table 4.1 Conditions that might be considered before diagnosing IBS *continued*

Condition	*Symptoms	*Tests
Eating disorders continued	Emotional instability	
	Damaged teeth	
	Reflux	
	Malnutrition	
	Bloating	
Microscopic colitis		
Microscopic inflammation of the bowel often associated with certain medications.	Watery diarrhoea that comes and goes	Colonsocopy
Laxative overuse/abuse		
A mental or physical reliance on laxatives that weakens the muscle tone of the gut. Long-term abuse can cause the gut to become sluggish and worsen chronic constipation.	Diarrhoea	Colonoscopy
	Constipation	
	Bloating	
	Wind	
	Nausea	
Urinary tract infection		
Bacterial infection in the bladder. Causes tiredness but a fever suggests a more serious kidney infection.	Painful urination	Urine test
	Smelly urine	
	Diarrhoea	

*Note: Not all symptoms may be present; and not all tests may need to be ordered.

The relationship between IBS and diet

Have you identified any foods or types of food that make the symptoms of IBS worse? For example, some people find that high-fat meals, caffeine (found in tea, coffee, chocolate and cola drinks), alcohol or spicy foods can make their symptoms worse. Often it is hard to identify one particular food that aggravates the problem—often it is hard to pinpoint any particular food that induces symptoms. Sometimes people with IBS can eat the same foods one day and not experience symptoms, then have almost exactly the same foods the next day and get symptoms. To help trace problem foods, keep a diary of the types of foods you have eaten the next time you have an attack of symptoms. Get in the habit of looking at the list of ingredients in processed foods to see if you can find a common ingredient that coincides with your attacks (e.g. onions).

Your doctor will want to see the diary and may refer you to a dietitian who will give you a dietary challenge (this is sometimes called an exclusion or elimination diet). This involves the dietitian identifying suspect foods in your diet that appear to worsen your IBS, and taking them out of your diet for a trial period of time (e.g. two to three months). Then, gradually over a number of weeks, your dietitian will ask you to reintroduce these foods into your diet to see if they make any difference to your symptoms. Depending on your lifestyle and other factors such as health and occupation, the dietitian might suggest taking the suspect foods out of the diet one at a time or all at once. The latter case can be quite extreme for some people and will not work with their lifestyle.

IBS and malabsorption

Relatively new research suggests that IBS can be triggered in some people by the malabsorption of certain short-chain carbohydrates (sugars) and polyols (sugar-free sweeteners). These sugars and sweeteners are often found in everyday products such as chewing gum, cordials, some yoghurt, stone fruits, kidney beans, chick-peas and milk.

Sue Shepherd, an Australian dietitian researching this area, has identified five dietary molecules as potential triggers for symptoms of IBS in people with visceral hypersensitivity. These are lactose (e.g. milk), sorbitol (e.g. stone fruit, artificial sweetener in chewing gum), fructose (apples and pears, and other specific fruits), raffinose (e.g. baked beans, cabbage), and fructans (wheat bread, onion, artichoke, asparagus). Together, these five dietary elements are called FODMAPs (fermentable oligo-, di- and mono-saccharides and polyols). Western societies are increasingly consuming large amount of FODMAPs, which may explain the rising incidence of IBS in these societies.

FODMAPs are poorly absorbed in the small intestine but highly fermentable in the large bowel, which means the sugars that are not absorbed in the small intestine pass into the large bowel. The large bowel is where normal bacteria in the bowel breaks down these sugars and sweeteners. This creates a problem because the bacterial action (fermentation) creates lots of gas, wind and bloating. In people with a hypersensitive bowel, the messages triggered by this fermentation activity are sent to the brain where they are interpreted as pain, and can also cause diarrhoea.

Check ingredient lists for these sugars and sweeteners, and avoid foods that contain them to see if it makes a difference to your symptoms. It is best to do this with the supervision of a dietitian. There are now books available (see end of chapter) that will tell you what supermarket food items contain FODMAPs.

Lactose intolerance

Some people may be just lactose intolerant. That is, they are born with insufficient amounts of the enzyme lactase, which is responsible for helping to digest lactose, the sugar in milk. All dairy products do not necessarily contain large amounts of lactose—for example, hard cheeses don't. With the guidance of your doctor or dietitian, try a low-lactose diet. If you find your symptoms are unchanged after a couple of weeks, there is no point in continuing and you should go back to your normal habit of drinking and eating milk products. Milk contains high levels of calcium, which are very important to bone fitness and reducing the risk of bowel cancer. If the non-dairy diet helps, ask your doctor or dietitian to check that you have enough calcium in your diet or to prescribe a calcium supplement. In some cases, people who have had a stomach or small bowel infection may have temporary lactose intolerance. If this has happened, try a lactose-free diet for six to eight weeks and see if it helps. Then gradually reintroduce milk products when you are feeling better. Soy products (with added calcium) can be a good source of calcium for people with lactose intolerance; however, sometimes soy-based foods can cause wind and bloating (from the soy beans).

Your doctor or dietitian will try to get a picture of your dietary habits that may be exacerbating your symptoms. For example, do you eat foods that are known to produce wind, such as lentils, beans, onions, artichokes, unripe bananas, leafy vegetables and cabbage? These foods could be making your problem worse. Also, did you know that some people who are badly constipated could get symptoms of diarrhoea? This is because when the bowel is blocked with faecal matter and the bowel has contracted many times trying to clear the blockage, some faecal fluid may ooze past, giving the impression of diarrhoea. This is called spurious diarrhoea or constipation with overflow.

Hydration

Your doctor or dietitian will also want to know if you are drinking enough water. Dehydration is a common cause of constipation. You should be drinking about eight glasses of fluids a day, and preferably water. Drinks such as tea, coffee and caffeinated sports drinks and alcohol can make dehydration worse because they are diuretics; that is, they make the kidneys produce more urine than normal. This means you are losing more fluid than you are drinking if you are not careful in choosing drinks wisely.

Fibre

Fibre is indigestible plant matter that is critical to our gastro-intestinal system. Fibre has many beneficial effects on the bowel and is an important factor in good digestive health. Generally fibre works by regulating the pace at which food moves through the gut. It slows down the pace of digestion when food is in the stomach. This is good because it makes you feel full and prevents overeating. It also slows down the release of sugars so that you have a more even sugar burst into your bloodstream, giving you energy for longer. Without fibre you get a hit of sugar that quickly comes and goes, which can leave you feeling tired and hungry sooner.

Further down the gut in the colon, fibre adds bulk to the waste products and helps stimulate a bowel motion. This is good because it prevents bad bacteria lingering in the bowel where they can produce lots of gas, causing discomfort and bloating. If you have diarrhoea, fibre can also sometimes help because it absorbs excess water and firms up the stool, also giving the gut wall time to rid the colon of fluid. Dietary fibre is also useful in reducing cholesterol blood levels by absorbing excess cholesterol. It is thought to aid good bacteria by working with them to produce a by-product that works like a natural antibiotic—defending the bowel from bad bacteria and protecting the gut wall from cancer. Foods that encourage the growth of good bacteria are known as **probiotics**.

Fibre comes in different forms that behave in different ways in our GIT. Types of dietary fibre include water soluble and insoluble. Lesser known forms are resistant starch and fructans.

Resistant starch and fructans resist digestion in the small intestine and are digested by the microflora (bacteria) in the large bowel. Resistant starch is found in legumes, bananas, cooled cooked potato, pasta, cornflakes and products made with 'Hi Maize'. Fructans are found in a few vegetables and plants, including wheat, onion, garlic, Jerusalem artichoke and chicory.

As normal bacteria break down these types of fibre in the large bowel and this fermentation process produces gas, resistant starch and fructans have important implications for people with IBS, with the possibility that they could make pain worse, as was discussed in relation to FODMAPs. This point will be returned to in a moment, but first, a little more about the differences between soluble and insoluble fibre and their beneficial qualities to health.

Soluble fibre is more readily broken down by normal bowel bacteria, while **insoluble fibre** is only slowly fermentable. Soluble fibre thickens food and slows down its passage in the digestive tract. Soluble fibre may also lower a food's GI rating.

GI stands for **Glycaemic Index** and refers to the measurement of how a carbohydrate food can affect the levels of glucose (sugar) in the blood. Low-GI foods raise the level of glucose in the blood slowly. Some diets focus on low-GI foods as a way of losing weight, by reducing sugar cravings because your blood sugar levels are under control. The lower the GI the better. This is because foods that cause a slower rise in blood sugar make you feel fuller for longer. For example, apples contain the soluble fibre pectin, which gives them a lower GI rating than watermelon, which has no pectin. Soluble fibre is also found in legumes (dried peas, beans and lentils), oats, barley and some fruits.

Insoluble fibre acts as a physical barrier to the digestive enzymes and slows down the digestive process. Insoluble fibres work like a sponge. They have waterholding properties in the large bowel and add bulk to the stool. They also bind cancer-causing molecules and bile acids to eliminate from the body. Foods such as 100 per cent bran breakfast cereals and whole grains are high in insoluble fibre. Foods containing cellulose or lignin, such as leafy vegetables and their stems, and wholegrain cereals and breads, contain good amounts of insoluble fibre.

If you need to increase your fibre intake, the type of fibre is important to consider, depending on what you want to achieve. If you need to lower cholesterol, or increase low-GI foods to control weight, soluble fibre, such as oat bran or psyllium, is better than insoluble. If you want to treat constipation, but want to avoid too much gas production, then insoluble fibre, such as sterculia, may be better. Always drink plenty of water with fibre—say 2 litres a day or more—to help your body cope with the increased load and improve its effectiveness.

For some people with IBS, increasing soluble fibre, resistant starch and fructans can increase gas production in the bowel, which can make pain and bloating worse. There are many studies currently being done to better understand the relationship of these types of fibres with IBS, and more research needs to be done before there is conclusive evidence. This is not a reason to remove fibre from the diet, but rather to try insoluble fibre or fibre supplements so that you are still getting the health benefits. Gradually introduce insoluble fibre into your diet over several weeks to give your bowel time to adjust to the increased levels. Your dietitian will be able to advise you as to what suits you best based on your symptoms.

Generally, if you have been diagnosed with IBS and suffer from constipation, it is recommended that you get between 25 and 30 grams of fibre each day. To give you a better idea, this is equivalent to two pieces of fruit *and* five serves of vegetables (half a cup if cooked, one cup if raw) *and* four serves of either bread, cereal, grain or pasta made from whole grains (a serve is one cup; a serve of bread is two thin slices).

It is very important to have enough fibre in your diet. Most Australians get less fibre than they should and this has been linked to Australia's relatively high rate of bowel cancer, diabetes, obesity and heart disease.

Lifestyle

IBS is more common in people with highly stressful lives arising from their jobs, home or study life. For more information on improving your lifestyle to help your digestive system, see chapter ten. But a few words here first. The key to improving your digestive health is reducing stress, increasing exercise, and identifying and stopping bad health habits such as smoking.

To change your lifestyle, you can help yourself by writing a list of all the things that you think are adding to the stress in your life and making changes where you can. If changing your job is out of the question, try to find more time to yourself during the working week. Can you take a walk at lunch? Can you walk to work, or park your car a little further from the office to give yourself some walking and thinking time before starting a busy day.

Exercise is a great buffer to stress. It increases the blood supply to our major organs, including the brain, and stimulates the release of happy hormones called endorphins. Think about increasing the amount of exercise in your week. Consider joining a gym, taking yoga classes, walking the dog, walking with friends after work, playing a team sport, riding a bike—the possibilities are many. Choose something you like and therefore will be able to stick with for the long-term.

Drugs

Medications can be very useful in treating IBS, but the types of drugs you may need will depend on your symptoms and their severity. These symptoms fluctuate; you may have good weeks and terrible weeks. You need to visit your doctor regularly so they can decide whether you need to adjust your medication to make sure you are getting the right doses when you need them. This means that you may not need the same medication long-term.

Below is a list of the major symptoms of IBS and the medications that can best help. But first, a note about drug side effects. Side effects can vary from individual to individual. Keep a note of what you are experiencing and when it started and be sure to tell your doctor. Some side effects are a nuisance while others are dangerous to your health, so your doctor needs to know about them. In many cases, side effects of drugs last no longer than a few weeks while your body is adjusting to the new drug so don't despair if at first you experience these unwanted effects, they may pass.

Abdominal pain

There are a number of medications available to help with some of the symptoms of IBS. Some drugs work by reducing spasm in the bowel, while others change the way the body interprets pain signals from the bowel. Some of these medications are also used as antidepressants, but for IBS these drugs are thought to work by a different mechanism of action by changing the way the body perceives pain.

Anticholinergic medications

Common anticholinergics that your doctor may prescribe are: Colofac, Buscopan and Atrobel. These drugs work by reducing bowel spasm. Be on the lookout for side effects, which may include a dry mouth and constipation.

SSRIs (selective serotonin reuptake inhibitors)

Common SSRIs that your doctor is likely to prescribe are fluoxetine and paroxetine. Side effects may include diarrhoea and restlessness. Do not take these drugs with other antidepressants or drugs such as Tramadol, which is a pain reliever.

Tricyclics

Tricyclics work much like SSRIs. Commonly used tricyclics include amitryptiline and dothiepin. Unwanted side effects may include drowsiness, low blood pressure and a dry mouth.

Other medications

Other medications that your doctor may prescribe include peppermint oil. For some patients, it has been found to help bloating and abdominal pain. Generally it does not have side effects.

Constipation
Stool-bulking agents
These are usually fibre supplements. Examples include Metamucil, Normafibre, Fybogel. These work by softening the stool and providing bulk. They need to be taken with plenty of water for maximum benefit. Just remember—those that are psyllium based (e.g. Metamucil) may cause bloating and excessive wind.

Laxatives
There are two main types of laxatives: osmotic and stimulant.

Osmotic laxatives work by drawing water from the body into the colon to soften the stool. Best taken with plenty of water, these are safe to use long-term. Examples include Movicol, Lactulose and Epsom salts. Unfortunately Lactulose can cause quite a bit of bloating: it is a type of sugar which is not absorbed by the small bowel but often fermented by bacteria in the large bowel instead, creating quite a bit of gas—something that is often not preferable for those suffering from constipation. Epsom salts is not only very safe but is also inexpensive, and is the authors' preferred choice when a laxative is required.

Unlike osmotic laxatives, **stimulant** laxatives are not recommended for long-term use. These drugs irritate the colon into action. As time goes on, larger doses are required for the same effect, to the stage where large doses of these laxatives are required just to maintain previous function. Examples of stimulant laxatives are Senna, Ford pills and Senokot. In some people, the effect of these drugs causes so much bowel irritation that it can make abdominal pain worse.

Also, increasing the amount of water or fluids you drink and regular exercise may help constipation, and is a great alternative to taking medications.

Other medications
Tegaserod was the first drug to be released specifically for the treatment of IBS—in particular, constipation-predominant IBS.

It works by decreasing the transit time of food through the bowel (reducing constipation) and by reducing the sensitivity of the bowel to being stretched—one of the major problems with IBS. Unfortunately the benefit seems to reduce over time and the drug is very expensive— at present it is not on the PBS (the government subsidised drug list). It is probably best used on a rotational basis with other strategies.

Diarrhoea
Antidiarrhoeal drugs

Not surprisingly these drugs slow the transit of food through the bowel, by acting on receptors in the bowel wall. Talk to your doctor before using them as they can be potentially dangerous when used during a bout of gastroenteritis or inflammatory bowel disease (IBD). Examples include Imodium, Loperamide and codeine phosphate. Loperamide and Imodium can occasionally cause a dry mouth. Antidiarrhoeal drugs are all safe to use long-term if necessary but they should not be used in children or elderly people unless directed by your doctor.

Cholestyramine

This drug is infrequently used for the treatment of diarrhoea. This medication binds bile salts which usually cause diarrhoea in those who have had previous bowel surgery, but sometimes it is beneficial in those who have IBS. It comes in sachets that are fairly unpalatable, and has been described as being like drinking concrete.

Non-drug treatments

In moderate to severe cases of IBS, the trigger may be more psychological than physical, and therefore it is important to understand if there are any underlying psychological disorders such as anxiety, sleep disorders, depression or psychiatric illness. Psychological disorders need to be treated separately to the IBS, and, where appropriate, your GP should refer you to a psychiatrist or psychologist trained to deal with these problems. Some IBS sufferers have improved greatly after undergoing therapies that promote coping techniques and relaxation, such as cognitive behaviour therapy, relaxation therapy and hypnotherapy. It is important to stress that many people who do not have an obvious psychological link to their bowel symptoms still often benefit from this approach.

Prognosis

IBS is a chronic condition with flare-ups and remissions. It often goes away after a while, but even if it doesn't, the right attitude—that means taking positive steps to improve your lifestyle—diet and medical help, can bring the disease under control so that you can get on with enjoying life. If you do not have an understanding GP or gastroenterologist, find one who is because this is the key to successfully managing your IBS. Fortunately IBS never leads to serious bowel disorders such as cancer.

Some common questions about IBS

My friend has IBS and she feels much better since going on a gluten-free diet. My GP has done a blood test for me for coeliac disease, which was negative. But I'm still feeling bloated and uncomfortable. Can I try a gluten-free diet too?

Yes. Many people find that they feel better on either a low-wheat or even gluten-free diet even if they do not have coeliac disease. In this situation it would be best to confirm that coeliac disease has been properly excluded, as occasionally the screening blood tests for coeliac disease can be falsely negative. In any case, wheat can be fermented by bacteria in the bowel creating gas, which can lead to abdominal pain and bloating. Foods that contain wheat often also contain quite a bit of fructans (made up from fructose units joined together). Some doctors and dietitians think that fructose malabsorption causes IBS in some IBS sufferers. Going on a low-fructose diet is worth considering. You should talk to your dietitian about this.

I am 36 and after confiding in a friend at work that I have IBS, I found that she does too. We both work in corporate finance. Is IBS more prevalent today than in my parents' generation?

Yes. There is no doubt that IBS is on the rise, particularly in developed nations. Whether that is because of better living conditions in general, a more stressful lifestyle, or changes in our diet is unclear. The most likely explanation, of course, is that it is a combination of all three. Many people in our parents' generation would also be less likely to seek or receive medical input should they have had IBS-type symptoms.

I am 29, pregnant with my first child and my IBS seems to be getting worse. Is this related to the pregnancy? What should I do?

IBS often gets worse during pregnancy. This is probably a result of hormonal changes along with the increased excitement associated with a new arrival. Many of the medications used in IBS are safe in pregnancy but, often, dietary changes, and in particular drinking more water, are good first steps. Check with your doctor before making changes to your diet during pregnancy.

After I told my doctor I had trouble sleeping and I have recently been divorced, she suggested I see a psychologist. I feel that she thinks the diarrhoea and constipation are problems of my mind and does not think IBS is a physical problem. Is IBS a label for something else?

No. IBS is a real condition that changes the way the bowel works. Scientific studies have shown that people with IBS have abnormal peristalsis (the coordinated contractions that move food along the bowel) and increased sensitivity to the bowel being stretched. Even though psychological factors can be an important component of IBS, they are not the full story.

I have had IBS for five years, should I be taking vitamins?

No. Although IBS can lead to diarrhoea, it does not affect the ability of the bowel to absorb nutrients or vitamins. As long as you eat a balanced diet, there is no need to take dietary supplements.

I have just been diagnosed with IBS and my doctor told me I have to change my diet. Do I have to give up alcohol?

Depends. People who consume a large amount of alcohol in one sitting (for example, binge drinking—say more than 60 ml of alcohol or six standard drinks) often complain of diarrhoea and abdominal pain for the next day or two. If binge drinking is a frequent occurrence, it can often be mistaken for IBS. However, some people find a small amount of alcohol helpful in IBS. If this helps you, a small amount—one to two standard drinks a day—shouldn't hurt.

My doctor gave me some Buscopan for some tummy pain, which helps, but I still get pain sometimes. What should I do next?

IBS is a chronic relapsing problem that requires a multi-pronged approach over a period of time. It could well be that additional strategies, such as lifestyle and dietary changes, may also help. It is important to realise that taking medication will not make it 'go away'.

A friend who works in a hospital told me that IBS is caused by spicy foods. Is this true?

No. Spicy foods definitely don't cause IBS. Some people may find that some spicy foods (for example, dahl) may trigger their symptoms; however, other components of the food (for example, lentils) are more likely to be the culprit and act as a trigger. Some foods can instead trigger reflux symptoms (in particular pastry, fatty foods and alcohol) that can be confused with IBS-type symptoms. If this is the case, then talking to your doctor or a dietitian who specialises in IBS may be helpful.

Further information

Medical contacts

Gastroenterological Society of Australia (GESA)
145 Macquarie Street
Sydney NSW 2000
Phone: (02) 9256 5454
Fax: (02) 9241 4586
Email: gesa@gesa.org.au
Website: www.gesa.org.au

British Society of Gastroenterology
3 St Andrews Place
Regents Park
London NW1 4LB
Phone: +44 (0) 20 7935 3150
Fax: +44 (0) 20 7487 3734
Email: bsg@mailbox.ulcc.ac.uk
Website: www.bsg.org.uk

American College of Gastroenterology
PO Box 342260
Bethesda, MD 20827-2260
Phone: +1 (301) 263 9000
Website: www.acg.gi.org

American College of Gastroenterology official patient information website: www.acg.gi.org/patients/patientinfo/ibs.asp.

IBS support groups

Irritable Bowel Information & Support Association of Australia (IBIS Australia)
PO Box 7092
Sippy Downs QLD 5456
Phone: (07) 3907 0527
Email: contact@ibis-australia.org
Website: www.ibis-australia.org

Irritable Bowel Syndrome Self Help and Support Group is an American support group that was established in 1987. Its website includes tips on managing the disease and personal anecdotes: www.ibsgroup.org.

The IBS Network is a UK charity established to help IBS sufferers: www. ibsnetwork.org.uk.

Books

2006 Fructose Malabsorption Food Product Guide
A handy pocket-sized guide with food product information and pictures telling you what foods contain FODMAPs and which brands are safe.
Author: Sue Shepherd
Publisher: Shepherd Works, 2006
Available at: www.coeliac.com.au

Conquering Irritable Bowel Syndrome
This book on IBS is written by arguably the world expert on the illness.
    Author: Nicholas Tally
    Publisher: BC Decker, 2005
    Available at: www.bcdecker.com

I.B.S. Relief
A doctor, a dietitian and a psychologist provide a team approach to managing irritable bowel syndrome.
    Author: Dawn Burstall, et al.
    Publisher: Wiley, 1998
    Available at: www.wiley.com

Irresistibles for the Irritable and *Two Irresistibles for the Irritable*
These two cookbooks by Australian dietitian Sue Shepherd provide recipes for anyone who needs a fructose-free diet or gluten-free diet or who is lactose intolerant.
    Author: Sue Shepherd
    Publisher: Shepherd Works, 2006
    Available at: www.coeliac.com.au

Wind Breaks: Coming to terms with wind
A light-hearted, but insightful book full of valuable information on flatulence, including its causes and how to treat it.
    Authors: Professor Terry Bolin and Rosemary Stanton
    Publisher: Margaret Gee Publishing, 1995
    Available at: www.amazon.com

Useful websites

The Australian Broadcasting Corporation has a health site with useful information and web links about IBS and other bowel disorders: www.abc.net.au/health/default.htm.

The Irritable Bowel Syndrome Association is an American self-help group that can be visited online at: www.ibsassociation.org.

Dietary information

To find an accredited dietitian in your state or territory, go to the Dietitians Association of Australia website. This site also has useful dietary tips and advice: www.daa.asn.au.

For tips on eating healthily and adding fibre to your diet, go to www.betterhealth.vic.gov.au.

An online information service set up by Australian gastroenterologists and health professionals includes dietary information for IBS and other digestive disorders: www.gastro.net.au.

5
Peptic ulcer disease

I have had a sensitive stomach during most of my adult years. I don't have time to go to the doctor so I take antacids and that seems to fix the problem for a while. But it always comes back. The pain is a gnawing, burning feeling and it gets worse when I eat. After a few hours it eases up until the next meal.

Stewart, 56, farmer

What is an ulcer?

An ulcer is a sore that forms in the lining of the stomach or the duodenum (the first part of the small intestine). It took the maverick Australian gastroenterologist Dr Barry Marshall and pathologist Dr Robin Warren to expose the great myth that ulcers were caused by stress or spicy foods. They discovered that ulcers were usually caused by an infection. They were able to prove that 70 per cent of stomach ulcers and 95 per cent of duodenal ulcers were caused by the bacterium, *Helicobacter pylori*.

Dr Marshall did this by swallowing the bacteria and developing severe stomach inflammation. Twenty years later, in 2005, they were jointly awarded the Nobel Prize in medicine for this important discovery.

Stomach and duodenal ulcers are commonly called **peptic ulcers**. Peptic ulcer disease is the term used when a person has been diagnosed with peptic ulcers.

Figure 5.1 A stomach ulcer

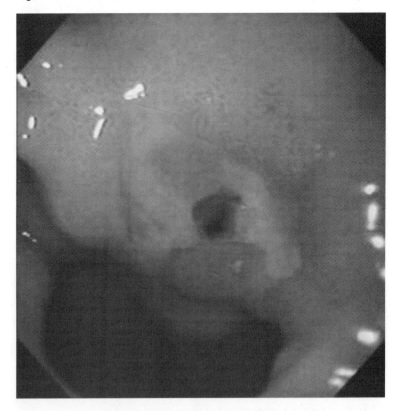

Who can get an ulcer?

An ulcer forms when the caustic effects of pepsin (an enzyme) and acid from the stomach's secretions overwhelm the body's natural defence mechanisms. *Helicobacter pylori* (*H. pylori*) changes the normal environment of the GIT by increasing the acid produced by the stomach and reducing defence mechanisms on the lining of the stomach. Normally, our bodies are designed to repel the damaging effects of stomach acid and pepsin. The lining of the stomach has a thin layer of mucus that keeps the acid and bacteria out. *H. pylori* changes this environment and makes it possible for ulcers to form.

We are all susceptible to *H. pylori* infection, but people from poorer areas or where lower levels of cleanliness or crowded living conditions exist are more vulnerable. These conditions make it easier for the bacterium to be passed from one person to another and this is why it is much more common in developing nations with poor sanitation. It has been estimated that more than half of the world's population is infected with *H. pylori*. But this does not mean that all those people go on to develop ulcers; usually other factors are involved (see below).

People of any age can get an ulcer, but it is rare to find children with ulcers. It is thought that children can acquire the bacterium but it is not until later in life that ulcers form. The bacterium remains in the stomach until treated. But while many of us may carry the bacterium, only a minority of infected adults go on to develop ulcers. It is thought that other conditions need to be present for an ulcer to form. These conditions might include genetic, immune or dietary factors.

Ulcers affect women and men equally. Government statistics record that about 500 000 Australians suffer ulcers at any one time. It is estimated that 10 per cent of Australians will suffer an ulcer at some time in their lives.

What else can cause an ulcer?

Apart from *H. pylori*, the most common cause of peptic ulcers is aspirin and non-steroidal anti-inflammatory drugs (NSAIDs). Other drugs such as steroids and chemotherapy can, less commonly, also cause ulcers. It is thought that 5 per cent of duodenal ulcers and 50 per cent of gastric ulcers are related to the use of NSAIDs. NSAIDs are very toxic to the lining of the stomach and can cause ulceration within half an hour of ingestion. NSAIDs damage the wall of the stomach directly, and also cause the stomach to stop producing acid. These drugs include aspirin, diclofenac (Voltaren), indomethacin (Indocid), naproxen (Naprosyn, Aleve), ibuprofen (Brufen, Nurofen, Advil, Nuprin, Rufen, Pamprin-IB), piroxicam (Feldene), and ketoprofen (Actron).

Regular users of these drugs are more likely to develop ulcers. One study estimated that between 15 per cent and 25 per cent of patients who have taken NSAIDs regularly had evidence of one or more ulcers, but in most cases the ulcers were very small. About 4 per cent of regular NSAID users went on to develop serious gastrointestinal conditions. Often, people who are at risk from developing ulcers, the elderly and the ill, are the same people who need to take NSAIDs regularly for chronic pain caused by inflammation. People at highest risk may be taking NSAIDs for conditions such as arthritis (particularly rheumatoid arthritis), chronic lower back pain, fibromyalgia, and repetitive strain injuries. People who also regularly take low-dose aspirin to prevent heart attacks are at even greater risk.

Other risk factors for developing an ulcer in NSAID users are:

- Aged over 65
- A history of peptic ulcers or upper gastrointestinal bleeding
- A history of heart disease or congestive heart failure
- Taking certain other medications such as anticoagulants like warfarin (Coumadin), corticosteroids, or the osteoporosis drugs alendronate (Fosamax) and risedronate (Actonel)
- Drinking alcohol
- Smoking
- Infection with *Helicobacter pylori*.

Newer anti-inflammatory drugs, such as celecoxib (Celebrex) and rofecoxib (Vioxx), have become available recently. Unfortunately, it seems that these drugs may increase the risk of heart attack, and should only be used short-term for people at low risk of heart trouble. The jury is still out on this, but currently it is recommended that people only take these drugs for short periods of time, and only if they are not at high risk of other medical problems such as heart disease or stroke.

Ulcers in severely ill patients

People who are severely ill in hospital are prone to getting ulcers because their immune system is in poor condition. The major concern here is that these ulcers may bleed. Patients, who are otherwise generally unwell, particularly in intensive care units (ICU), can develop so-called 'stress ulcers'. These are usually only superficial, but can be widespread throughout the stomach. Patients at risk of stress ulceration are given medication to prevent it. Patients who are most likely to gain from this prophylactic treatment are:

- People with serious burn injuries—greater than 30 per cent of their body
- Very ill patients with blood-clotting problems
- People being treated in an ICU who need a ventilator for more than two days.

Is peptic ulcer disease inherited?

Studies have found that if one identical twin has an ulcer, the other is likely to develop one too. Early studies also found an association between certain blood groups and ulcers. People who have an immediate family member with an ulcer are also thought to be at higher risk. But whether the risk is higher because of environmental factors, such as exposure to *H. pylori*, or genetic factors is difficult to say conclusively. Some researchers think there is a genetic predisposition but no particular gene has been found to be responsible for people developing ulcers. This question is still being investigated.

How do you know you have an ulcer?

The signs and symptoms of an ulcer can vary depending on where the ulcer is in the GIT. Many people with peptic ulcers have no symptoms whatsoever, but the commonest symptoms are pain and nausea. The pain is usually described as a 'burning sensation' or 'gnawing' and is felt in the middle of the abdomen, under the ribs, called the **epigastrium**. It can travel between the ribs or to the back. The pain can cause sufferers to wake up in the middle of the night. It can last for days or even a few weeks. Rarely, an ulcer can cause vomiting.

People with a duodenal ulcer may find that the pain disappears when they eat. For this reason, they may put on weight because eating becomes a way to ease pain. The opposite sensation happens to people with stomach ulcers. Eating can make the pain much worse. Some people might self-medicate with over-the-counter tablets that reduce the acidity of the stomach, which can make the ulcer feel less painful because it is not being aggravated by the acid. But treating the pain will not make the ulcer go away. In fact, a history of taking these tablets to relieve abdominal pain is itself an indication that an ulcer may be present.

Complications of peptic ulcers

When ulcers are left untreated there can be complications. However, complications are rare because ulcers are easily diagnosed and treated by doctors. When complications do arise they are: bleeding, perforation, obstruction, anaemia and cancer.

Bleeding and perforation

Two serious complications of peptic ulcers are bleeding and perforation. Both can be life-threatening events. Bleeding is when the ulcer erodes a nearby blood vessel causing internal bleeding.

Perforation involves the space next to the GIT called the **peritoneal cavity**. If the ulcer is deep enough, it erodes through the wall of the stomach or duodenum and breaks through to the peritoneal cavity, allowing gastric contents to flow into this area. This is called a **perforation** and it usually causes sudden, sharp and severe pain. In 10 per cent of perforations, bleeding internally also occurs.

When an ulcer bleeds or perforates, the patient usually lies still from the pain, and is obviously distressed. Their pulse rate and breathing quicken. Their abdomen may become hard and feels very sore when touched.

Perforated and bleeding ulcers need to be treated straightaway. If a lot of blood is lost, the patient may need a blood transfusion. The ulcer may need surgery to stop the bleeding and to repair the perforation. These days most bleeding ulcers can be treated without surgery by using a gastroscope. A skilled practitioner can insert a device into the gastroscope to inject drugs or a hot coil of wire to stop the bleeding by burning the blood vessel; this is called **cauterisation** or **diathermy**.

Obstruction

Long-term inflammation from an ulcer can cause swelling and scarring. This can block the outlet of the stomach and stop food from passing into the small intestine. This can lead to vomiting and abdominal pain. Previously, this condition always required surgery, but new anti-ulcer medications can often remedy this without an operation. Occasionally the narrowing can be dilated endoscopically through a gastroscope, using a special balloon.

Anaemia

A bleeding ulcer can cause a fall in your red blood cells, which contain haemoglobin, the compound that transports oxygen in the bloodstream to your body. With too little haemoglobin, you may feel the effects of anaemia, which are tiredness, feeling the cold, increased breathing and pulse rate, and poor memory. Depending on how low your red blood cell levels are, your doctor may suggest you take iron tablets for a short time until the levels are restored. In serious, but rare, cases the levels may be very low because of a big bleed and a blood transfusion may be needed.

Cancer

Occasionally peptic ulcers can actually be a form of cancer. This is very uncommon. In a small number of patients, studies have found that severe *H. pylori* infection goes on to develop into stomach cancer. A biopsy should be done when an ulcer is first diagnosed to rule out this rare complication.

Diseases associated with ulcers

Some long-term illnesses have been associated with peptic ulcer disease. Ulcers have been found in one in three patients with chronic lung disease; the reasons why are unclear, but it may be related to cigarette smoking or steroid use.

People with cirrhosis of the liver are also at a higher risk of getting an ulcer. It is thought that people who suffer hardening of the heart's blood vessels or hormonal conditions, such as

Cushing's disease, and hyperparathyroidism may also be at higher risk, but no studies have been able to produce solid evidence to confirm this suspicion.

How is an ulcer diagnosed?

An ulcer cannot be properly diagnosed without tests. But before your doctor orders any of the tests below, they will want to ask you some questions; this is called taking a personal history. Also, they will probably want to do a general physical examination.

Personal history

Taking your history is a way for your doctor to get to know you and find out relevant medical information about you that may help them to pinpoint the problem. A history usually involves asking questions about family, physical health, social, dietary and psychological aspects of your life. To help your doctor make a correct diagnosis, you should volunteer any information that you think may be helpful. Generally, they are likely to want to know about your symptoms, when they are at their worst, and if anything you do relieves them, such as taking medication or eating food. It is vital that your doctor is aware of all medications you are taking. This is particularly important as some drugs can be linked to the cause of ulcers. They may also ask questions about your bowel actions and dietary habits.

Physical examination

Most doctors will want to do a general physical examination to make sure there are no obvious problems that have been missed. This will involve routine health checks such as measuring your blood pressure. This is a painless and quick procedure that involves placing a cuff around your arm that is attached to a sphygmomanometer. They may also want to check your mouth for ulcers, and listen to your heart and lungs with a stethoscope by placing it on your chest and on your back. Your doctor may feel your abdomen to check for tenderness when touched or for abnormal swelling.

Tests

All or some of the following tests may be ordered. (For more information on tests, see chapter two.) The main reasons are to see if an ulcer can be sighted and if the bacterium *H. pylori*—the most common cause of ulcers—can be found:

- **Endoscopy with biopsy (gastroscopy)**—The gastroscopy will take around five minutes and is usually done under sedation by a gastroenterologist. It involves inserting a thin flexible telescopic tube into the mouth and down into the oesophagus, stomach and beginning of the small bowel (duodenum). The gastroenterologist will look for an ulcer in the stomach and duodenum, and for other possible causes to account for the symptoms, such as gastro-oesophageal reflux disease (see chapter six). If an ulcer is found, they should take a biopsy to send to the laboratory to see if *H. pylori* is present. The patient usually has no memory of the procedure and suffers no pain or discomfort.
- **Radiography (barium swallow and/or barium meal)**— This test is rarely used these days because endoscopy is the test of choice, usually. Unlike endoscopy, a doctor cannot take a biopsy using this method. But, if a patient has complicated ulcer disease, very occasionally this test may be ordered to have a good look at the stomach and duodenum. It involves swallowing barium, a non-toxic white, chalky-tasting fluid, and then taking an X-ray. The barium fills the stomach and small intestine, and allows the X-ray to make

a picture of these structures which will show any ulcers if present.

- **A stool sample**—You may be asked to provide a sample of your stool to be sent to the laboratory to check if you have any blood in it caused by a bleeding ulcer. You may not be able to physically see the blood but, if tiny amounts are there, the test will pick it up. Large amounts of blood usually change the colour of the stool from brown to black. Blood in the stool also makes it smell more pungent. Stool samples can also be used to test for the presence of *H. pylori.*

- **Blood test**—A sample of blood may be taken from your arm to test for the presence of *H. pylori.* Your doctor may also test your iron levels: if your ulcer has been bleeding, they could be low.

- **Urea breath test**—This test involves breathing into a bag (like an alcohol breathalyser). It is ordered if there is a chance that *H. pylori* is present but wasn't found by the other tests (this can be called a false negative). This can happen if the patient has used antibiotics or other drugs that treat ulcers within the previous two weeks. It is also a safe test for children and pregnant women. It is also a useful test to see if *H. pylori* has been successfully eradicated.

If it is not an ulcer, then what?

The main feature of peptic ulcer disease is abdominal pain. Some of the other conditions that can be confused with this pain are listed in the table on page 112. A peptic ulcer cannot be diagnosed accurately on symptoms alone. It is very important that a doctor assesses any abdominal pain. Your doctor may suspect an ulcer based on your symptoms, but only tests can confirm the diagnosis.

Table 5.1 Diseases that can have similar symptoms to a peptic ulcer

Condition	*Symptoms	*Tests
Inflammatory bowel disease (IBD) IBD includes ulcerative colitis and Crohn's disease. IBD is a chronic illness with inflammation of the bowel. See chapter eight for detailed information.	Abdominal pain Diarrhoea Blood and mucus in stools Weight loss Tiredness Anaemia Skin and eye problems Wind Bloating	Colonoscopy Barium X-ray Blood tests
Non-ulcer dyspepsia Abdominal pain like ulcer pain but with no obvious physical cause.	Repeated episodes of upper abdominal pain or discomfort Fullness Symptoms may be related to meals, overeating or stress	Gastroscopy Blood tests
Medication side effects	Abdominal pain Wind Bloating Diarrhoea or constipation Vomiting and nausea Reflux	Endoscopy Blood tests

Table 5.1 Diseases that can have similar symptoms to a peptic ulcer
continued

Condition	*Symptoms	*Tests
Cancer of the pancreas	Abdominal pain	CT scan
	Weight loss	Ultrasound
	Jaundice (yellow skin)	
Pancreatitis		
Inflammation of a gland that makes enzymes for digestion and also insulin. Often caused by gall stones or alcohol.	Severe abdominal pain Vomiting Sometimes jaundice (yellow skin)	Blood tests CT scan Ultrasound
Gall stones		
Only cause trouble when they are blocked in the gall bladder or bile duct and cause an obstruction.	Episodic abdominal pain Sometimes jaundice (yellow skin)	Blood tests Ultrasound
Reflux disease (see chapter six)		
When stomach secretions backflow into the gullet and cause health problems.	Heartburn Regurgitation Waterbrash (excess saliva) Chest pain Nausea Hoarseness Cough Sore throat Difficulty swallowing	Endoscopy

*Note: Not all symptoms may be present; and not all tests may need to be ordered.

Treating ulcers

The good news is that most ulcers can be treated with drugs. In severe cases, surgery is necessary to sew over the ulcer to stop it bleeding; however, this is uncommon. In very severe cases, the stomach may need to be taken out: this is very rare since the advent of modern medication, and is therefore not something most people need to worry about. The typical treatments for ulcers are outlined below.

Medication

As most ulcers are caused by *H. pylori,* ulcer treatment is focused on getting rid of this bad bacterium from the GIT. This is done with antibiotics. As well as the antibiotics, medication may be prescribed to help ease the pain and heal the ulcer. This is called **antisecretory therapy**. These tablets work by reducing the acidity of the stomach. Less acid means less aggravation to the ulcer and less pain.

If the ulcer is believed to be caused by taking tablets such as the NSAIDs listed previously, these should be stopped immediately if possible. People with severe arthritis or heart conditions may need to continue with their drugs, especially aspirin. If this is your situation, you need to discuss treatment options with your doctor.

Eradication therapy for H. pylori
This usually involves a pack of drugs called Nexium Hp7 which is taken for one week. It contains: Nexium 20 mg, to be taken twice a day; the antibiotic Amoxil 1 g, twice a day; and Clarithromycin 500 mg, twice a day.

Antisecretory therapy
Either of two types of tablets can be given to reduce the acid in the stomach. They are proton pump inhibitors (PPIs) or histamine

H2-receptor antagonists (H2RAs). The rate of healing is often faster with PPIs. PPIs include lansoprazole, omeprazole, pantoprazole and rabeprazole. H2RAs are generally not used these days, as PPIs are so much more effective. H2RAs include cimetidine, famotidine, nizatidine and ranitidine.

Generally, antisecretory therapy should involve taking tablets for between four and eight weeks to give the ulcer a chance to heal. For more information about the individual PPIs and H2RAs, see chapter six.

Other medications

If you have experienced a bleeding ulcer, your iron levels may be low and your doctor may want you to take supplementary iron. This is a tablet, usually taken once a day. It can cause constipation, so be sure to drink plenty of water and make sure there is enough fibre in your diet.

Diet

No study has found a convincing link between diet and peptic ulcer disease.

However, some people find that certain foods and drinks can upset their stomach (called **dyspepsia**). This is a different issue and dyspepsia can be dealt with by avoiding those substances (see chapter six for more information on diet and dyspepsia).

Tea, coffee, cola soft drinks and decaffeinated versions of tea and coffee can stimulate the secretion of gastric acid, but again there have been no studies that have found these drinks increase the likelihood of developing an ulcer. Interestingly, studies that looked at the effects of bland diets on ulcer disease also found no evidence that it helped. In fact, some bland foods stimulated a considerable amount of acid secretion.

Lifestyle

There is no strong evidence that emotional stress causes ulcers, but it probably does cause the symptom, dyspepsia. Therefore lifestyle changes will make little difference to established ulcer disease. The main causes are the bacterium *H. pylori* and non-steroidal drugs (NSAIDs). The important thing is to stop taking NSAIDs under your doctor's supervision and to treat the *H. pylori*, if it is present, with antibiotics as prescribed.

Surgery

Surgery is necessary for a small minority of patients who have life-threatening complications of peptic ulcer disease, such as haemorrhage, perforation, penetration or obstruction (see pages 106–7). Not all patients with a bleeding ulcer will need surgery. The type of surgery depends on the size and position of the ulcer and health of the patient. It is more likely to be necessary in an emergency situation, such as a life-threatening perforation, rather than as an elective procedure.

Prognosis

Mostly, the prognosis for peptic ulcer disease is excellent. Most ulcers can be cured with tablets alone. Recurrence is unlikely once the cause of the ulcer—usually *H. pylori* or NSAIDs—has been eradicated from the body. In very few people, who usually need to take NSAIDs or have other health problems, recurrence can occur. They will need to be monitored by endoscopy and may need to be treated with long-term antisecretory therapy as prescribed by their gastroenterologist. As discussed above, surgery for the treatment of ulcers is very uncommon.

Repeat gastroscopies are usually only performed to document

the healing of gastric ulcers, and to exclude the possibility of cancer.

Some common questions about ulcers

I work in the reception of a busy city law firm and have recently been treated for a gastric ulcer. My aunty told me that ulcers are related to emotional stress, but my doctor hasn't mentioned this. Is it true?

No, stress does not cause ulcers. Ulcers are caused by infection with the bacterium, *Helicobacter pylori*, or by taking non-steroidal anti-inflammatory drugs (NSAIDs). However, recent research has suggested that some people infected with *H. pylori* are more susceptible to getting ulcers than others. Emotional stress has been raised as one of many factors that might increase the risk of being infected with *H. pylori*, but this has yet to be proven.

I have been diagnosed with a stomach ulcer. Are there certain foods or drinks that I should avoid?

Not really. Food generally doesn't cause ulcers; however, some foods may make your symptoms worse. If this is the case, then they are best avoided. Foods that commonly make symptoms worse can be spicy foods. Also, excessive amounts of alcohol may prevent ulcers from healing as well.

Does alcohol or smoking cause ulcers?

Alcohol and smoking probably cause a very small proportion of ulcers, and certainly can delay healing. If you smoke and also have an ulcer, it may be a good opportunity to stop smoking!

My wife was treated for a stomach ulcer and was due to have a follow-up endoscopy, but she has just found out that she is eight weeks pregnant. Is it safe to have the procedure and should she stop taking her antisecretory tablets?

This would depend on the location and severity of the ulcer. In most cases, the follow-up endoscopy could be delayed until after delivery of the baby; however, you should check with your doctor. Some newer ulcer drugs are generally not used in pregnancy as there is more safety data supporting the use of the older drugs such as ranitidine (Zantac).

My doctor said I had a peptic ulcer in the stomach. I have been reading about ulcers and am confused about the difference between a peptic ulcer, a gastric ulcer and a duodenal ulcer.

Gastric and duodenal ulcers are both types of peptic ulcers. A gastric ulcer is found in the stomach and a duodenal ulcer is in the first part of the small intestine.

If ulcers are caused by an infection, does this mean they are contagious?

Most peptic ulcers are caused by an infection with bacteria called *Helicobacter pylori.* This can be spread from person to person but most people who get infected pick it up during childhood. Infection is thought to be passed on in the household; for example, on chopsticks, cutlery and toothbrushes.

I have read that the probiotics in foods like yoghurt are very good for stomach problems. Would these probiotics help heal my stomach ulcer?

Probiotics are becoming increasingly popular and seem to be particularly good for preventing travellers' diarrhoea. Currently there are no probiotics available for the treatment of peptic ulcers, and, due to the hostile environment in the stomach, it is probably unlikely that one will become available soon.

Is there a vaccine for peptic ulcers?

A vaccine is being developed, but as yet there is no commercially available vaccine. Scientists have successfully developed a vaccine for animals. Human trials are underway.

Further information

Medical contacts

Gastroenterological Society of Australia (GESA)
145 Macquarie Street
Sydney NSW 2000
Phone: (02) 9256 5454
Fax: (02) 9241 4586
Email: gesa@gesa.org.au
Website: www.gesa.org.au

British Society of Gastroenterology
3 St Andrews Place
Regents Park
London NW1 4LB
Phone: +44 (0) 20 7935 3150
Fax: +44(0) 20 7487 3734
Email: bsg@mailbox.ulcc.ac.uk
Website: http://www.bsg.org.uk

The **American College of Gastroenterology** official patient information website: www.acg.gi.org/patients/patientinfo/ulcers.asp.

Useful websites

An online information service set up by Australian gastroenterologists and health professionals includes dietary information for IBS and other digestive disorders: www.gastro.net.au.

The Medical Journal of Australia website has some good articles on peptic ulcer disease. This site is better suited to health professionals who are familiar with medical language: www.mja.com.au.

National Digestive Diseases Information Clearinghouse (NDDIC) is a website that discusses peptic ulcers and explains how *H. pylori* can cause them. It also provides information on diagnosis and treatment: www.digestive.niddk.nih.gov/ddiseases/pubs/hpylori/.

This American government health website by the Centers for Disease Control and Prevention provides an easy-to-understand guide to peptic ulcer disease. It also has a searchable database of articles on peptic ulcer disease: www.cdc.gov/ulcer/.

The man who discovered *Helicobacter pylori*, Dr Barry Marshall, set up the *Helicobacter pylori* Foundation in 1994. The foundation's website includes frequently asked questions, useful links and on-line discussion: www.helico.com.

6
Reflux disease

Six months ago I got a promotion at work. Since then I have been working longer hours and am often living on takeaway food eaten just before going to bed. I gained five kilos and my heartburn is terrible—I chew on Rennies all day. One of the senior partners at work had heartburn and ended up dying from cancer of the gullet. I'm frightened I might end up the same way. I need to do something about this.

Peter, 45, accountant

What is reflux disease?

Reflux disease is very common in Western societies, and it's on the rise. It can affect anyone—young or old—causing symptoms such as heartburn and indigestion . . . There are actually two types of reflux disease, but first we will discuss what reflux is.

Reflux

Reflux occurs when some of our stomach contents enter the oesophagus (gullet). It can be a normal phenomenon, and usually happens shortly after eating.

Normally, the stomach contents are kept separate from the oesophagus by a ring of muscle, the lower oesophageal sphincter (LOS). When the LOS does not close properly, for whatever reason, the stomach contents, which are usually acidic, can backflow into the oesophagus causing reflux.

The body has ways to protect itself from the damaging effects of reflux. When we are upright during the day, gravity stops the reflux from travelling up the oesophagus. Also, we regularly swallow and this helps wash reflux back into the stomach. Saliva is slightly alkaline and this can neutralise the effects of acidic reflux. During sleep, we can be more susceptible to reflux because we are lying down and no longer have the advantage of gravity to stop the stomach's contents going up the oesophagus. But, generally, other factors need to be present for reflux to be a problem, such as a hiatus hernia or a poorly functioning LOS.

Reflux disease

Reflux disease is when the refluxed fluid, which contains acid and pepsin (an enzyme that begins the digestion of proteins) produced by the stomach, causes health problems. There are two forms of reflux disease: gastro-oesophageal reflux disease (GERD or GORD) and non-erosive reflux disease (NERD).

People are diagnosed with GERD when the exposure of the oesophagus to the stomach's contents causes erosion of the oesophagus, which can be seen on endoscopy. **Oesophagitis** is a widely used term to describe inflammation or damage of the oesophagus.

People diagnosed as suffering NERD (some doctors don't differentiate and call this GERD too) have reflux disease symptoms but show no physical evidence of erosion of the oesophagus.

In fact, most people with reflux disease do not have visible ulceration when their oesophagus is examined by endoscopy. Only about one-third of patients with reflux disease have evidence of oesophageal erosion.

Reflux disease is not an easy disease to define. This is because symptoms are varied, and they can be vague, having different meanings to different people. For example, what someone describes as chest pain, someone else may call heartburn. Also, many healthy people experience symptoms such as heartburn without suffering reflux disease. About 20 per cent of adults in Western society experience heartburn at least once a week. Often, this occurs after drinking more alcohol than usual or eating certain foods that bring on heartburn attacks.

At the other end of the spectrum, GERD can be a very serious condition that can be life threatening. In people with chronic GERD, it can cause a change in the appearance of oesophageal cells, known as **Barrett's oesophagus**. In very few people, GERD is thought to lead to cancer of the oesophagus—but it must be stressed that the risk of this is very small.

What are the symptoms of reflux disease?

As there is no universal agreement on what defines reflux disease, doctors need to take a careful history and examination to identify symptoms. The more common symptoms are heartburn (pyrosis), acid regurgitation, and difficulty swallowing (dysphagia). Many people with reflux disease may describe any or all of these as 'indigestion'. This is a general term for a stomach upset that may be accompanied by discomfort, heartburn or nausea.

Heartburn

When doctors talk about heartburn, they are referring to a burning sensation behind the breast plate (sternum) that comes from the top of the abdomen (epigastrium) and may radiate towards the throat. It can come and go, and usually occurs within one hour of eating, while lying flat or during exercise.

Heartburn is often relieved by drinking water or taking a tablet or liquid that neutralises the acid, called an **antacid**. Almost everyone experiences heartburn from time to time, but when symptoms occur frequently and interfere with your lifestyle, it is termed reflux disease. That said, not all people with reflux disease experience heartburn.

Acid regurgitation

This is when the stomach's contents, or bile, has travelled back up into the stomach from the duodenum (the first part of the small intestine) and continues up the oesophagus to the throat (pharynx) without causing nausea or retching. Those who experience regurgitation may describe a sour or burning fluid in the throat or mouth that can contain bits of food. It can be made worse by bending, burping or any activity that raises the pressure in the abdomen.

Dysphagia

This term describes difficulty swallowing. People with dysphagia complain that food won't go down properly and it may feel like it sticks in the throat. Less commonly, they may complain of throat pain. It is a symptom that should not be ignored and often indicates serious reflux disease. About one-third of people with reflux disease complain of dysphagia. The causes can be mechanical, such as a narrowing of the oesophagus caused by scarring, inflammation of the oesophagus, or faulty peristalsis—the wave-like movements of the oesophagus that send food down to the stomach. Dysphagia can also be due to abnormal sensitivity to the movement of food bulk during peristalsis.

Other symptoms

Less common symptoms of reflux disease include: the excessive production of saliva called **waterbrash**; excessive belching; queasiness; and nausea. Some people may complain of a cough that won't go away, especially a dry cough in the morning; bad breath; asthma; or a hoarse voice. Others may experience severe pain on swallowing called **odynophagia**. This is often caused by something other than GERD, such as infectious oesophagitis, and should be investigated for other causes. Another symptom of reflux disease is chest pain—this should always be investigated to rule out heart complications.

Table 6.1 Summary of reflux disease symptoms

Common	Less common	Needs to be treated promptly
Heartburn	Chest pain	Dysphagia
Regurgitation	Nausea	Coughing up blood (Haematemesis)
Waterbrash	Hoarseness	Weight loss
	Cough	Sore throat

Who gets reflux disease?

Unfortunately, it is very common in Western societies. Reflux disease is the most common cause of heartburn and indigestion. It can affect anyone including infants, children and pregnant women. In America, the United Kingdom, Canada, Australia and most Western countries, reflux disease is an expensive problem, costing billions of health dollars and many sick days from work every year. A recent Australian study found that up to two million adult Australians suffered heartburn that interfered with their sleep for up to an hour a night, three nights a week. The study's authors estimated that many of these people called in sick to work because they were tired from lack of sleep due to reflux symptoms. Sydney University Associate Professor Martin Weltman, a gastroenterologist, commenting on the study, told the media: 'Frequent heartburn can severely impact quality of life and productivity of sufferers'. He said heartburn was often mistakenly trivialised, when in fact it affects one in five Australians and can cause serious complications if not treated properly.

In the United States, it is estimated that 95 million adults suffer some sort of digestive problem and more than 61 million adult Americans suffer reflux at least once a month.

Generally, those at higher risk of reflux disease are smokers, people who drink alcohol (more than seven standard drinks a week), anyone with an immediate family member diagnosed with reflux disease, and people suffering obesity.

Also at higher risk are people diagnosed with medical conditions such as connective tissue disease, asthma or cystic fibrosis. And, it is more common in people who are institutionalised because they can spend long periods of time in bed.

Research has found that Anglo-Saxon populations are more affected by GERD than other races. Women and men are equally affected (but men are twice as likely to get oesophagitis and Barrett's oesophagus). Interestingly, people with the bacteria that cause ulcers, *Helicobacter pylori*, are generally **less likely** to suffer reflux disease than the normal population. This inverse relationship is complex and not well understood.

Usually, reflux disease is a long-term problem. Symptoms may be mild and come and go. In more severe cases, symptoms can occur daily. Most people suffering reflux disease need long-term management with medication.

What causes reflux disease?

Reflux disease results after frequent reflux episodes. Reflux episodes usually happen because the LOS is not closing properly and therefore allows the acidic stomach contents to backflow into the oesophagus. Some things make reflux worse, but this depends on the individual. Foods and drinks that are known to lower LOS pressure, allowing reflux to occur, include foods high in fat, chocolate, caffeine and alcohol, as well as some drugs. Cigarettes also decrease LOS pressure and can make reflux worse.

Reflux disease can also be made worse when the pressure in the abdomen is raised. This can happen if you are overweight. Losing weight can improve reflux symptoms.

In pregnancy it is thought that hormones and the increased abdominal pressure caused by the growing foetus make the LOS less effective.

Hiatal hernia (or hiatus hernia) is also common in reflux disease and often blamed for it, although its occurrence does not necessarily mean reflux disease is present. A hiatal hernia occurs when part of the stomach protrudes through the oesophageal opening of the diaphragm, which can alter the abdominal pressure and stop the sphincter closing properly.

Reflux in children

Regurgitation and vomiting are common in infants less than six months old. Usually it improves with age. If the child appears otherwise well, and there is no associated irritability or high temperature (greater than 37.5 degrees Celsius), there is no need to worry. Often the baby will be keen to feed again immediately after vomiting. If the baby is calm, there is no reason not to continue feeding on the baby's demand.

Figure 6.1 No hiatal (hiatus) hernia

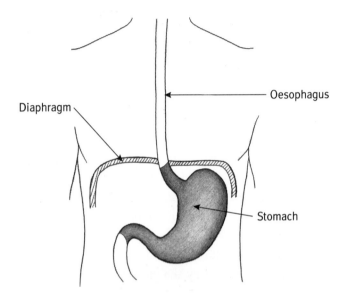

Figure 6.2 Hiatal hernia present

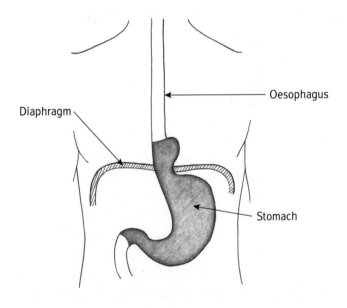

Simple measures can be used to help the baby with reflux, such as putting them on their side when feeding. Also, the head of the cot or basket can be raised to use gravity to help keep milk down. In newborns, over-the-counter treatments such as Gripe water and Infacol can help—always check the directions first and the recommended minimum age.

In older babies, usually after four months, feeds can be thickened to help prevent reflux—check with your doctor if your baby is less than four months old. This can be done by adding half to one teaspoon of maize-based flour to the boiled water used for making the formula. In breast-fed babies, the thickening agent can be added to breast milk and given by bottle.

Less commonly, vomiting and regurgitation may be a symptom of other conditions. If the vomiting persists and the baby looks unwell, is dehydrated, has a high temperature, or does not want to feed or play, see your doctor immediately.

Complications of reflux disease

Barrett's oesophagus

A rare complication of reflux disease can be a change in the cells lining the lower end of the oesophagus. This condition is called Barrett's oesophagus and, although rare, it is thought to be a cause of oesophageal cancer. It is found by endoscopy in up to 10 per cent of patients with longstanding reflux disease. Most people with Barrett's oesophagus go undiagnosed.

People found to have Barrett's oesophagus should have a biopsy taken to rule out cancer. They require follow-up endo-scopies and biopsies every five years. Because the risk of cancer is so low, at this stage, medical experts do not think it is worthwhile screening all patients who have reflux for Barrett's oesophagus.

It would be very costly and cause unnecessary distress to patients who are otherwise well.

Cough and asthma

Reflux is an irritant to the nerves of the oesophagus. Some of the messages that go to the brain from these nerves trigger us to cough. Reflux can be a cause of a chronic unexplained cough. It can also be one of the many irritants that trigger asthma in people who are prone to it.

Asthma is the narrowing of the tubes in the lungs, which can make it difficult to breath. The air becomes trapped in the lungs making it more difficult to breathe out. Asthmatics wheeze when they breathe out because the air is trying to get out of a constricted space. It is a potentially life-threatening condition and needs to be **properly** and **promptly** managed by a doctor.

Sore throat and pneumonia

If refluxed liquid gets past the upper oesophageal sphincter (UOS), it can enter the throat (pharynx) and the voice box (larynx). This causes inflammation that can produce a sore throat and hoarseness. Refluxed liquid that passes the larynx can also enter the lungs. This can lead to an infection of the lungs such as pneumonia. It is a serious problem and needs urgent treatment, usually in hospital.

Strictures

Repeated exposure to acidic reflux in the oesophagus can cause scar tissue that can narrow the gullet. This is a stricture. Strictures are rare in reflux disease. In people with oesophagitis, the incidence of strictures ranges from 8 per cent to 20 per cent.

The danger of strictures is that they can increase the risk of food getting stuck and cause choking. But, since the widespread use of proton pump inhibitors (PPIs), the prevalence of strictures is decreasing. Similarly, bleeding from the oesophagus is now uncommon, occurring in less than 2 per cent of patients.

Treatment of strictures

Strictures are easily treated at endoscopy by dilatation with either a balloon or bougie (a soft plastic tube). This procedure can cause some mild discomfort afterwards, which generally settles down. Very rarely it can lead to a split in the lining of the oesophagus. In extremely rare cases, the stricture may need surgery.

Adenocarcinoma

Adenocarcinoma is a type of cancer of the oesophagus that usually occurs near the junction between the stomach and oesophagus. Although never proven, it is thought that reflux disease and Barrett's oesophagus may go on to develop into adenocarcinoma in some people. This condition is becoming more common in the Western world. It sounds odd but this is possibly because of better conditions and the widespread use of antibiotics that have made the bacteria that causes stomach ulcers, *Helicobacter pylori*, less common. Research suggests that this bacterium, while a cause of ulcers, can reduce acid secretion in the stomach, and reduce the prevalence of reflux in the community.

How is reflux disease diagnosed?

Reflux disease can have very similar symptoms to other GIT problems. Diagnosis is usually based on symptoms and on your doctor taking a thorough medical history.

The most common symptom is heartburn but, as mentioned earlier, this can mean different things to different people. It is best described as a 'burning feeling rising up from the stomach or lower chest towards the neck'.

Unlike many conditions, the severity of the symptoms does not reveal the severity of the reflux disease. If your doctor suspects reflux disease based on your symptoms, they may start you on a two-week trial of a drug that reduces stomach acid secretion, called a proton pump inhibitor (PPI). After taking the medication, people with reflux disease should start to improve quickly. In this instance, endoscopy is NOT necessary.

Further investigations are needed when the diagnosis remains unclear and symptoms do not disappear, or if complications are suspected, or if alarm symptoms are present, such as painful swallowing, coughing up blood, choking attacks (especially at night), or unexplained weight loss. Tests may include those listed below.

Endoscopy (gastroscopy)

The gastroscopy will take around ten minutes and is usually done under sedation by a gastroenterologist. It involves inserting a telescopic tube into the mouth and down into the oesophagus, stomach and beginning of the small bowel. The gastroenterologist will look for signs of reflux disease in the oesophagus and other possible causes of symptoms in the stomach and duodenum, such as an ulcer. They may take a biopsy. However, it is important to realise that more than half of patients with reflux symptoms will have a **normal** endoscopy result and there is no point taking a biopsy in these patients.

Video capsule endoscopy

This test has been traditionally used to look at the small bowel, but is now available to look at the oesophagus. It involves the patient swallowing a tiny pill-sized camera, which transmits a video to a small receiver, a bit bigger than a mobile phone, worn on a belt. The doctor reviews the video at a later date. Although very expensive, this test takes only one minute, and requires no special preparation or an anaesthetic.

pH monitoring

If endoscopy and a trial of medication were unsuccessful in finding the problem, your doctor may order 24-hour ambulatory oesophageal pH monitoring. This involves passing down the nose, a very fine tube that is connected to a small box, like a digital camera. The tube measures the amount of acid present in the oesophagus over 24 hours. It is generally only used in difficult cases and for people contemplating surgery.

Barium swallow

This is not a common test for diagnosing reflux disease because other tests are better. But, it is useful for assessing patients who have difficulty swallowing caused by a stricture.

Manometry

This test is done rarely but is useful when there is a problem with the coordination of muscle contractions in the oesophagus that can cause trouble swallowing (dysphagia) and pain on swallowing (odynophagia). Manometry involves placing a slim tube, which measures the pressure in the oesophagus at various levels, down through the nose. It is particularly useful for diagnosing achalasia.

If it is not reflux disease, then what?

There is much overlap between the symptoms of reflux disease and other GIT disorders. About two-thirds of patients who report upper abdominal pain or discomfort also complain of reflux symptoms. Table 6.2 (see page 136) lists some of the suspected conditions that may be investigated before a diagnosis is made.

Treating reflux

In treating reflux disease, your doctor is aiming to improve your quality of life by relieving symptoms, healing the inflamed oesophagus (where this is the case), and reducing the risk of complications. Treatment can include lifestyle and dietary changes, medications and surgery.

Lifestyle changes

For people with mild or occasional reflux symptoms, lifestyle changes, and occasional use of over-the-counter antacid tablets when pain is present, may be all that is needed. Changes that may help are listed below.

Lifestyle changes
Do

- Elevate the head of the bed if you have symptoms at night. To cause less disruption to partners, a wedge pillow may be more practical.
- Cut back on alcohol, particularly red wine. The low pH of red wine (or any alcoholic drink) can make reflux symptoms worse.
- Check with your doctor if you are on other medications. Some drugs make reflux symptoms worse. These include some heart tablets, drugs used to treat Parkinson's disease, aspirin and anti-inflammatory medications.
- Watch your weight. Being overweight can be a risk factor for reflux.
- Add fibre to your diet to avoid straining when you go to the toilet because this can increase intra-abdominal pressure and make reflux worse (e.g. wholegrain breads and cereals, more fruit and vegetables with the skins left on).

> **Don't**
>
> • Eat large meals, or eat late at night.
> • Lie flat shortly after meals—allow at least two to three hours after eating before going to bed.
> • Wear tight-fitting clothes, especially after meals.
> • Smoke—smoking makes reflux worse and increases the risk of cancer of the throat and oesophagus.

Dietary changes

Some foods make reflux worse. These vary from person to person. Keep a diary of what you eat and make a note of which foods seem to make your symptoms worse. Take these out of your diet, one at a time, where possible and see if it makes a difference. Anecdotal evidence suggests that citrus fruits, tomato products, spicy foods and carbonated drinks can make reflux worse by inducing symptoms in people with oesophagitis. Try and introduce these foods again at a later date to see if you can tolerate them. It is important to avoid unnecessary food restrictions. Also, try not to be too strict with your diet or you will find it hard to stick to it.

Drugs

There are two groups of drugs used to treat reflux disease: prescription drugs and over-the-counter drugs. Generally, prescription drugs are more powerful, but may have more serious side effects. The various drug options belonging to the two groups are explained below.

Over-the-counter medications
As the name suggests, these drugs do not require a prescription and can usually be bought from pharmacies and supermarkets.

Table 6.2 Conditions that might be considered before diagnosing reflux disease

Condition	*Symptoms	*Tests
Peptic ulcer disease		
A break in the lining of the stomach or duodenum.	Abdominal pain Nausea Vomiting	Gastroscopy
Non-ulcer dyspepsia		
Pain similar to that of an ulcer caused by spasm or stretching of the stomach.	Abdominal pain Bloating Nausea	Gastroscopy Blood tests
Irritable bowel syndrome (IBS)		
Abnormal sensitivity and coordination of muscle contraction in the bowel.	Abdominal pain Nausea Bloating Diarrhoea Constipation	Gastroscopy Colonoscopy Blood tests
Achalasia		
Severe spasm of the lower oesophagus.	Severe pain Dysphagia	Gastroscopy Manometry
Coronary heart disease		
Narrowing of the arteries around the heart—can include a 'heart attack'.	Chest pain especially on exertion	ECG Coronary angiogram Exercise test
Biliary colic		
Pain caused by a gall stone blocking the neck of the gall bladder.	Episodic abdominal pain with vomiting	Ultrasound
Oesophageal spasm	Pain on swallowing Dysphagia	Gastroscopy Manometry

*Note: Not all symptoms may be present; and not all tests may need to be ordered.

These drugs include antacids and a group of drugs called histamine H2-receptor antagonists (H2RAs). They work by reducing the amount of acid in the stomach. Antacids include Mylanta, Gaviscon and Rennie. They account for more than one billion dollars in sales per year in the United States.

Histamine H2-receptor antagonists are sold under the trade names of Zantac, Pepcidine and Gaviscon Advance. They should only be used for the relief of mild and occasional reflux symptoms. If you are regularly self-medicating—more than twice a week—it is time to see your doctor to get more effective treatment. This is important because regular use of these drugs will NOT heal oesophagitis and complications can arise.

Prescribed drugs

Your doctor's aims in prescribing medication for reflux disease are: to confirm the diagnosis by seeing if the symptoms clear up; to give relief from symptoms; and to heal oesophagitis, if present.

The prescribed drugs fall into two categories: proton pump inhibitors and prokinetics.

Proton pump inhibitors (PPIs)

- *What are they?*—These tablets work not by preventing reflux from occurring, but by reducing the acid in the reflux so that less irritation occurs.
- *How do they work?*—These tablets stop acid production in the stomach by acting directly on the pump mechanism in the stomach's parietal cells, which make acid.
- *Examples of PPIs*—omeprazole (Losec), lansoprazole (Zoton), pantoprazole (Somac), rabeprazole (Pariet), esomeprazole (Nexium).
- *How long will I need to take them?*—Generally, these tablets are used for six weeks and then the dose is 'stepped down' to the minimum dose needed to control symptoms.

- *Are there side effects?*—Generally none at all, but rarely they can cause mild diarrhoea, and interact with other tablets such as Warfarin, a blood-thinning tablet. PPIs have been used for more than 20 years without any long-term side effects.

Prokinetics

- *What are they?*—These tablets speed up the emptying rate of food leaving the stomach, which means there is less content to reflux.
- *How do they work?*—They act on the stomach's nerve supply by increasing the signals to empty the stomach.
- *Examples of prokinetics*—metoclopramide (Maxolon), domperidone (Motilium).
- *How long will I need to take them?*—These tablets can be used for as long as needed, but are usually prescribed long term.
- *Are there side effects?*—These tablets are not suitable for children. Very rarely they can cause painful spasms of the back muscles, called an oculogyric crisis.

Surgery

Surgery is very rarely required these days for reflux. The most common procedure done is called a **Nissen fundoplication**. This is done through laparoscopic (keyhole) surgery and is generally reserved for people with debilitating symptoms that cannot be controlled by medication. Before considering surgery, it is important to have manometry and pH testing to be sure that there is not another reason for the drug treatment not working, such as achalasia—a disease of the muscle of the oesophagus—or another motility problem. The surgery involves wrapping part of the stomach around the bottom end of the oesophagus to help prevent stomach contents from coming up and causing reflux. This surgery is very effective; however, if it is done too tightly, occasionally people have trouble swallowing after the procedure, but this can be fixed.

Prognosis

Recent studies have shown that most people with symptomatic reflux disease wait one to three years before getting medical help. It has also been found that the severity of the disease is not related to the duration of symptoms. Most people with reflux disease respond well and can be symptom-free on long-term medication. Less severe cases may require medication infrequently.

People who suffer severe oesophagitis are less fortunate, and are likely to have flare-ups every now and then. One study showed more than 80 per cent of chronic sufferers had recurrent oesophagitis after discontinuing medication. For this reason, long-term use of medications is generally recommended.

Barrett's oesophagus is an uncommon complication of reflux disease, but it is more common in men than women; some studies suggest it is ten times more likely in men. Recent studies suggest that obese Anglo-Saxon males with reflux symptoms were most at risk of oesophageal cancer resulting from reflux disease. And, although the risk is small, this type of cancer is on the increase in the United States and other Western nations. But, even among the high-risk group, the chance of developing oesophageal cancer was less than a one in two thousand. Although it has never been proven, it is thought that staying on treatment for reflux disease prevents Barrett's oesophagus from progressing to cancer.

Among reflux disease sufferers who have had a laparoscopic Nissen fundoplication, more than 90 per cent of patients reported no reflux symptoms after the procedure.

Some common questions about reflux disease

I work night shift and have been drinking a lot of coffee to stay alert. Recently I have had chest pain. When I wake up from sleep I often have a sore throat. My doctor couldn't find any heart problems and said I probably had reflux disease. How did I get this?

You have probably had reflux for some time, which has been made worse by difficult sleep patterns and drinking more coffee. Trying to reduce your coffee intake and avoiding food and drink before sleeping may help, but medications, and possibly an endoscopy, may be required.

My daughter is six months pregnant and has terrible heartburn. What can she do to treat it? Will it lead to anything more serious?

Heartburn during pregnancy is so common that it is almost expected. Antacids and ranitidine are both safe in pregnancy and are usually all that is required. It will settle down once the baby is born. It is unlikely to have any long-term consequences.

I have had heartburn for years. A friend with a similar problem said that she had reflux disease. What is the difference between heartburn and reflux disease?

This is a tricky question. Heartburn is a symptom of reflux disease. We define reflux disease as symptoms such as heartburn that occur frequently enough to interfere with one's lifestyle, generally more than twice a week. You have reflux disease if you are getting heartburn this regularly.

My husband has been diagnosed with a hiatus hernia. I read an article about reflux disease and it mentioned hiatus hernia as a cause. I wondered what is the difference between reflux disease and a hiatus hernia?

A hiatus hernia is usually caused by the stomach 'sliding up' above the diaphragm (see Figure 6.2, page 128). Although it does not cause reflux disease, it does make reflux more likely to occur—the diaphragm usually helps to keep the lower oesophageal sphincter shut.

I have bad heartburn and a friend suggested I avoid spicy foods and fat? Is this an old wives' tale?

Studies have shown fatty foods, alcohol and caffeine all loosen the lower oesophageal sphincter, which is the cause of reflux. Some people notice other foods, like spicy foods and onions, do the same. If a particular food always worsens your symptoms, try taking it out of your diet for a trial period of six to eight weeks—it could improve your reflux symptoms.

I have just been diagnosed with reflux disease, then I read that it can lead to cancer of the oesophagus and I am now petrified. Is this true?

Although it has never been proven that reflux disease causes cancer of the oesophagus, it probably does happen but is extremely rare. Everybody experiences reflux from time to time but very few of these people have ulceration in the oesophagus and hardly any of these ever go on to get cancer. Sometimes an endoscopy is performed, to exclude Barrett's oesophagus or cancer; generally this is done in people who have a new onset of symptoms after the age of 50, or troublesome symptoms that are not responding to treatment.

When I get heartburn, it seems to make my asthma worse. Why does this happen?

There is no doubt that reflux can be a cause of asthma due to chemical irritation of the lungs with acid. This usually responds very well to treatment with PPIs.

Is there a cure for reflux disease?

No. Most people find satisfactory relief with medication such as PPIs and need to take drugs only occasionally after an initial course of treatment is finished. Although surgery is available, most people don't need it and prefer taking occasional medications.

Further information

Medical contacts

Gastroenterological Society of Australia (GESA)
145 Macquarie Street
Sydney NSW 2000
Phone: (02) 9256 5454
Fax: (02) 9241 4586
Email: gesa@gesa.org.au
Website: www.gesa.org.au

American Gastroenterological Association (AGA)
National Office
4930 Del Ray Avenue
Bethesda, MD 20814
Phone: + 1 (301) 654 2055
Fax: +1 (301) 654 5920
Email: member@gastro.org
Website: www.gastro.org

American College of Gastroenterology official patient information website: www.acg.gi.org/patients/patientinfo/gerd.asp.

British Society of Gastroenterology
3 St Andrews Place
Regents Park
London NW1 4LB
Phone: +44 (0) 20 7935 3150
Fax: + 44 (0) 20 7487 3734
Email: bsg@mailbox.ulcc.ac.uk
Website: www.bsg.org.uk

Support groups

You can see what other GERD sufferers have to say at one of the many online chat rooms. This site offers helpful dietary tips and advice: www.heartburn.about.com/od/supportgroups/.

PAGER (Pediatric Adolescent Gastroesophageal Reflux Association) is an American not-for-profit organisation that provides useful information to parents who have children who suffer reflux: www.reflux.org.

Dietary contacts

Australia
The Gut Foundation is an Australian organisation that provides professional and public education, and promotes research into digestive disorders to improve gastrointestinal health: www.gut.nsw.edu.au.

You can also find a qualified dietitian in your state or territory by visiting the **Dietitians Association of Australia** website. This also has useful dietary tips and advice: www.daa.asn.au.

Britain

British Nutrition Foundation is a scientific and educational charity that promotes the wellbeing of society through nutritional knowledge and advice: www.nutrition.org.uk.

CORE (was Digestive Disorders Foundation) is a UK site that provides fact sheets on reflux disease. Contact them at:
3 St Andrews Place
London NW1 4LB
Phone: +44 (0) 20 7486 0341 (this is not a helpline)
Fax: +44 (0) 20 7224 2012
Email: info@corecharity.org.uk
Website: www.corecharity.org.au

Patient UK is a directory of UK health websites that provides information fact sheets written by doctors on many health topics including acid reflux and oesophagitis: www.patient.co.uk.

United States of America

This government-run website is all about diet and nutrition. You can learn how to maintain a healthy weight to reduce the risk of reflux disease: www.healthierus.gov/nutrition.html.

Books

Gastrointestinal Nutrition: A comprehensive guide to the dietetic management of conditions of the gastrointestinal tract
As its name suggests, this Australian book, written by two dietitians, is about a range of GIT conditions including reflux disease. It is aimed at health professionals but is a terrific book for understanding about nutrition and the GIT and includes some practical advice.
Authors: Amanda Anderson and Sue Shepherd
Publisher: Monash Medical Centre (Southern Health), 2003

How to Stop Heartburn: Simple ways to heal heartburn and acid reflux
This book provides advice on managing heartburn. Its co-author Dr Anil Minocha is the Professor of Medicine and Director of the Division of Digestive Diseases at the University of Mississippi Medical Center in Jackson, USA.
    Authors: Anil Minocha and Christine Adamec
    Publisher: Wiley, 2001

Heartburn and Reflux for Dummies
Carol Ann Rinzler, a medical writer, and Dr DeVault have teamed up to write about all aspects of heartburn and its treatment.
    Authors: Carol Ann Rinzler and Ken DeVault
    Publisher: For Dummies, 2004

Useful websites

The Gastroenterological Society of Australia has provided an information leaflet on heartburn that can be downloaded free at: www.gesa.org.au/leaflets/heartburn.cfm.

A New Zealand website, sponsored by the Gastric Reflux Support Network New Zealand for Parents of Infants and Children Charitable Trust (GRSNNZ), provides information to parents who have children that suffer from reflux: www.cryingoverspilt milk.co.nz.

A UK website on digestive disorders, set up by the National Health Service (NHS), has many links to other UK resources: www.equip.nhs.uk/topics/digest.html.

A US government website provides information about digestive diseases: National Digestive Diseases Information Clearinghouse (NDDIC) http://digestive.niddk.nih.gov/ddiseases/pubs/gerd.

Another US health website brings together information from America's National Institutes of Health (NIH) and other government agencies and health-related organisations: www.nlm.nih.gov/medlineplus/gerd.html.

7
Coeliac disease

I work at a bank in the city. Two years ago I was told by my GP that I have irritable bowel syndrome after suffering many years of abdominal cramps, bloating and sometimes diarrhoea; particularly when I get stressed. Six months ago I 'cracked a rib' while coughing, which led to my doctor organising bone density testing. It showed I had thin bones and I was referred to an endocrinologist (hormone specialist) who discovered I have coeliac disease. Since going on a gluten-free diet and taking calcium and vitamin D supplements, I now feel less tired, my diarrhoea has disappeared, I no longer get stomach cramps and my ribs have healed.

Siobhan, 27, bank lender

What is coeliac disease?

Coeliac disease (pronounced seel-ee-ak) is a permanent intestinal intolerance to dietary gluten. In untreated coeliac disease, the lining of the small bowel (intestine) is damaged. The disorder mainly affects the small bowel and is caused by the body reacting to ingested wheat gluten or related proteins found in rye, barley, triticale (a hybrid of wheat and rye) and oats. Wheat has the highest concentration of gluten and does the most damage to the lining of the small intestine, which is covered in finger-like structures called villi. It is the job of villi to absorb nutrients. Most forms of wheat, including durum, semolina, spelt, kamut, einkorn and faro, contain gluten that damages the villi in people with coeliac disease.

In persons with coeliac disease, the villi often appear shrunken and flattened compared to the small intestinal lining of persons without the disease. People with coeliac disease are less able to absorb nutrients from the small intestine than people with normal villi. Rye, oats and barley contain less gluten than wheat; however, ALL gluten causes damage.

Figure 7.1 An endoscopic view of a healthy duodenum

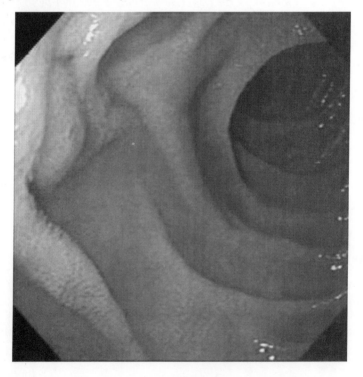

Figure 7.2 Flattened villi due to coeliac disease

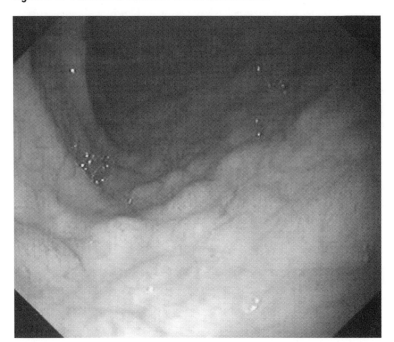

People affected by coeliac disease usually have a genetic predisposition to it. This means it may be partially inherited. A family history of coeliac disease puts you at a greater than average risk of suffering the disease. The cause of coeliac disease is complex, with multiple factors involved, but research suggests the gene, human leukocyte antibody (HLA)-DQ2, is strongly associated with the disease.

History of coeliac disease

Aretaeus the Cappadocian first detected the condition in the first century CE. It wasn't until the Second World War that the link between diet and the disease was confirmed, when Willem Karel Dickie, a Dutch paediatrician, found that wheat worsened the condition. During the war, the wheat flour used to make bread was scarce. Children suffering coeliac disease appeared to improve during this time of rations. After the war, when the cereal supply was replenished, the children with coeliac disease relapsed.

Over the years, coeliac disease has been described by various names. The technical term for coeliac disease is **coeliac sprue**. The English spelling of the disease is *coeliac,* compared to the American spelling of *celiac*. Other terms for the condition have included nontropical sprue, coeliac syndrome, adult coeliac disease, idiopathic steatorrhoea, primary malabsorption, wheat allergy and gluten insensitivity.

Who does coeliac disease affect?

Statistics on the incidence of coeliac disease do not reflect the incidence in Australia. It used to be quoted that about one in two thousand Australians had coeliac disease, but some doctors and dietitians working in the area now think it is more likely to be one in a hundred. Some of the reasons for the great disparity in these numbers is that many more Australians than have been identified are thought to suffer the disease and have not been correctly diagnosed because their symptoms are absent or subtle. Some people don't experience symptoms of the disease until adulthood. Others have symptoms in childhood that may disappear during adolescence and may or may not return later in life.

If you have a first-degree relative (i.e. mother, father, brother, sister) with coeliac disease, the likelihood of developing the disease is increased to one in ten. The condition is twice as common in women as men.

Coeliac disease is associated with other conditions and diseases. Data that was studied during the decade of 1990 to 2000, in which coeliac disease was positively identified by blood test and biopsy, found that the diseases that had an association with it included: early onset insulin-dependent diabetes mellitus, hypothyroidism, epilepsy in children, primary bilary cirrhosis, lymphoma of the gastrointestinal tract, Addison's disease, and chromosomal disorders such as Down syndrome and Turner syndrome.

Coeliac disease is more prevalent in some countries than others. Studies into the geographical incidence of the disease have found that it is high in Western Europe and it is more common in Celtic populations. It is also very high in Italy, Sweden and the south-east of Austria. Places where Europeans have emigrated, such as Australia and America, have a similar incidence rate of the disease.

The condition is not limited to Caucasians. Studies in the UK have shown coeliac disease is now as common among West Asian immigrants in England as its Caucasian population.

The condition has been reported in other national populations including Sub-Saharan Africans, Arabs, Hispanics, Israeli Jews of European heritage, Sudanese of mixed Arab-African descent, and Cantonese. However, the condition rarely, if ever, affects people of purely Chinese or Japanese descent.

The reasons for the difference in incidence rates between different cultural and racial groups are not fully known, but a large part of it is understood to be genetic. As stated earlier, the prevalence of coeliac disease among first-degree relatives is about 10 per cent. Studies have shown that the likelihood of an identical twin having coeliac after the other has been diagnosed is about 70 per cent, suggesting that genetic factors play a major role in determining the disease.

But other factors, such as the timing of the introduction of gluten into a child's diet, the differences in gluten protein concentration in various infant formulas, and the subjective nature of interpreting small intestinal biopsies to diagnose coeliac disease, are also believed to play a role in the varying incidence rates.

What causes coeliac disease?

The short and less complicated answer is gluten. More specifically, the proteins in gluten—glutenin and gliadin—cause the body to react against itself through an immune response that damages the lining of the small intestine. In rye, the damaging protein is called secalin; in barley, it is hordein; and in oats, it is avenin. In turn, this affects the body's ability to absorb vital nutrients. Deficiencies in some of these nutrients can cause other serious health problems.

However, as noted earlier, the causes of coeliac disease are multifactorial with diet, genetics and the immune system playing a role.

How do you know you have coeliac disease?

The symptoms of coeliac disease can vary from person to person, which can make diagnosis difficult. The most common symptoms are associated with the small intestine's inability to do its job properly, causing nutrient malabsorption. These symptoms include: tiredness or lethargy, diarrhoea, abdominal pain, flatulence, bloating and indigestion. However, because of greater awareness of coeliac disease, more accurate testing and screening of relatives, people are being diagnosed earlier, before they display the more severe signs of the disease. Fifteen years ago, people with coeliac disease may have experienced episodic diarrhoea with more than ten stools a day. These stools may have been light in colour and greasy, both signs of stearrhorea (fat in the stool): fat was not being absorbed properly. These symptoms are not so commonly seen today. This is because the disease is better understood and detected earlier by doctors before the villi are significantly damaged.

Occasionally, some people have none of the more common gastrointestinal symptoms and instead go to their doctor with associated diseases or complications, such as osteoporosis—loss of calcium causing weakness in the bones. Another non-gastrointestinal condition associated with 10 per cent of coeliac patients that also responds to a gluten-free diet is the auto-immune disease known as **dermatitis herpetiformis**, which causes a rash over the body.

Other presentations of coeliac disease can be blood deficiencies, such as in iron, vitamin D, zinc folate and vitamin B12.

Some general symptoms that may be caused by coeliac disease include:

- Loose stools
- Poor weight gain
- Vomiting
- Apparent food intolerances
- Other gastrointestinal symptoms (e.g. reflux)
- Mood swings
- General weakness.

Children and coeliac disease

In children, the typical symptoms begin shortly after the child has been weaned off breast milk, or cereals are introduced into the diet. Symptoms may include pale-coloured, smelly stools; occasional crampy, abdominal pain; or discomfort with or without vomiting.

The child may fail to thrive and suffer muscle wasting, or abdominal distension, and may have watery diarrhoea with occasional constipation. Their mood may be apathetic and irritable.

In older children, anaemia and nutritional deficiencies may be present. In rare cases, but still seen in some Asian children, rickets (a vitamin-D deficiency that, in extreme cases, causes weak, bent bones, particularly of the legs) may be obvious. Often, coeliac disease may disappear during adolescence.

But, as with adults, some children with coeliac disease may not have any obvious symptoms. For this reason, coeliac disease should be tested for in children that are failing to thrive who have an ethnic background at greater risk of the disease. Short children who are diagnosed with coeliac disease and begin a gluten-free diet before puberty often catch up to other children with a growth spurt.

Why it is important to diagnose—complications

Don't be tempted to self-diagnose. Gimmicky products such as 'wheat sensitivity tests' purchased over the Internet cannot give a definitive diagnosis one way or the other. To find out if you have coeliac disease, you will need to see a doctor to have a blood test and probably a gastroscopy—a scope that goes down the mouth, down the oesophagus and stomach, and into the small intestine to look at the intestinal lining.

It is important to diagnose coeliac disease if it is present so that the damage to the intestinal lining can be stalled or reversed by starting a gluten-free diet. Also, because coeliac disease affects the absorption of vital nutrients and minerals, running low on these elements can affect parts of the body other than the digestive system.

If not diagnosed, adults with coeliac disease are, on average, seven centimetres shorter than their peers. This does not mean that tall people do not suffer coeliac disease. In severe cases, tall people with the disease may be very underweight and may have signs of muscle wasting.

Without diagnosis and treatment, complications of coeliac disease include: blood deficiencies; damage to the neurological and skeletal systems, causing muscle weakness, unsteadiness and bone pain; menstrual abnormalities in women; and infertility or lowered fertility in both sexes. While coeliac disease sufferers are not renowned for having psychological abnormalities, many who start a gluten-free diet report a vast improvement in their mood and reduction in irritability and depression.

How is coeliac disease diagnosed?

To diagnose coeliac disease, your doctor needs to take a thorough medical history—including asking about family members and whether they have been diagnosed with coeliac disease or other auto-immune diseases such as dermatitis herpetiformis, insulin-dependent diabetes, thyroid problems and osteoporosis. They will do a physical examination that may involve feeling your abdomen to rule out other causes, as well as general health checks such as taking your blood pressure and testing your reflexes. To confirm a diagnosis, your doctor will need to order blood tests and a gastroscopy and small bowel biopsy. Patients should also be encouraged to have a bone density scan to see if osteoporosis is present.

Tests and investigations may include the following. However, not all of these tests may be necessary for you. The tests ordered would depend on the symptoms you present with.

Blood tests

Your doctor should order blood tests. The newest blood test now widely available is called **EMA**, which stands for serum endomysial autoantibodies. It is highly specific and a big improvement on the previous blood tests for coeliac disease. It can detect if your body has reacted to gluten by producing anti-bodies. The presence of the antibodies usually suggests coeliac disease. It is possible that the test can be occasionally falsely negative, in which case a biopsy of the small intestine will confirm diagnosis.

Also, your doctor should take blood to check for anaemia and any deficiencies, especially in folic acid, iron, vitamin D and vitamin B12. They may also want to check your calcium levels to rule out other complications.

A gastroscopy with biopsy

The gastroscopy will take around ten minutes and is usually done under sedation by a gastroenterologist. It involves inserting a telescopic tube into the mouth, down the oesophagus into the stomach, and then down into the small bowel. This allows the gastroenterologist to see the tissue in the small bowel and to observe any obvious abnormalities. The biopsy will be taken from the small bowel using a long instrument like tweezers, which is inserted inside the gastroscope. This is a painless procedure because of the lack of nerve endings in the surface tissue of the small bowel. The biopsy is sent to the laboratory, where a pathologist will look at the tissue under a microscope to check if there is any damage or abnormalities with the cells of the small bowel. If the disease is present and obvious, the gastroenterologist will be able to see the flattened villi at the time of the test. Both the blood antibody tests and gastroscopy must be done while gluten is still part of the diet otherwise the tests may appear normal.

Bone density test

If you have been diagnosed with coeliac disease in adulthood, you should have a bone density test to assess the calcium levels in your bones. It is a painless procedure and is similar to a simple X-ray. It usually involves lying still on a table while an overhead machine scans the bones. It takes about five to ten minutes.

Stool examination

This is very rarely done, but may be ordered if you have a lot of pale, offensive-smelling stools (due to possible fat malabsorption). It involves collecting your stools in a container for up to three days. The stools are sent to the laboratory where the fat content is analysed.

Diseases associated with coeliac disease

Dermatitis herpetiformis (DH)

Dermatitis herpetiformis, also called Duhring's disease, is a rare gluten-sensitive blistering skin condition that is very itchy, even in the presence of a mild rash. The rash is typically found over the kneecap, on the outer surface of the elbows, on the buttock area, around the ears, the shoulderblades, and in the hairline and eyebrows. It tends to be fairly evenly spread on both sides of the body. When the rash subsides, which it often does spontaneously, it may leave brown pigmentation or pale areas, where pigmentation is lost. The rash typically consists of raised lesions similar in appearance to herpes (hence the name), but it is not related to the herpes virus. It is not contagious. It can look like small insect bites with tiny fluid-filled blisters. In some people, the lumps are more like hives, or it can be pink and scaly like dermatitis.

The rash can come and go without treatment. If it is not treated, dermatitis herpetiformis can run a very long course, over many years—sometimes improving, sometimes getting worse—but it may go away eventually. The rash is usually treated with an antibiotic called dapsone and a gluten-free diet. Very occasionally, dapsone can have side effects including causing a fall in the red blood cell levels. This is usually dose related and your doctor may monitor your red blood cell count with regular blood tests. A lukewarm bath followed by an anti-itch lotion containing menthol or phenol can help relieve the pain.

Insulin-dependent diabetes mellitus (IDDM)

Coeliac disease affects 5 per cent of people with IDDM, and it should be routinely checked for in everyone with IDDM. This is because coeliac disease can make it more difficult to control blood sugar levels, along with other problems. Also, long-standing diabetes can affect the movement of the small and large bowel. This can cause diarrhoea at night, alternating with constipation.

Lymphocytic colitis

Lymphocytic colitis is a microscopic inflammation of the bowel. It is a common cause of watery diarrhoea in older people—most people are diagnosed in their 60s or later—and sometimes it can be related to coeliac disease. It is usually diagnosed by taking a biopsy during colonoscopy. If you have lymphocytic colitis, it is important to rule out coeliac disease as a gluten-free diet can improve symptoms of this condition.

If it is not coeliac disease, then what?

Coeliac disease can mimic many other diseases because it can cause trouble with many areas of the body and be difficult to pick up. Irritable bowel syndrome (IBS) can be impossible to distinguish from coeliac disease just from the symptoms alone. Table 7.1 shows some of the other conditions your doctor may want to investigate based on the symptoms that are also common to coeliac disease.

Table 7.1 Conditions that might be considered before diagnosing coeliac disease

Condition	*Symptoms	*Tests
Irritable bowel syndrome (IBS)		
increased sensitivity of the bowel to being stretched or problems in the way the bowel moves food along.	Abdominal pain Bloating Diarrhoea and/or constipation	Blood tests Gastroscopy Colonoscopy
Non-ulcer dyspepsia		
Pain similar to that of an ulcer caused by spasm or stretching of the stomach.	Abdominal pain Bloating Nausea	Gastroscopy Blood tests
Dietary deficiency		
Not enough iron, B12 or folate in the diet (vegetarians particularly susceptible to vitamin deficiencies if diet is not balanced).	Tiredness Fatigue	Blood tests
Inflammatory bowel disease (IBD)		
Inflammation of the bowel wall.	Abdominal pain Diarrhoea Rectal bleeding Tiredness Weight loss	Gastroscopy Colonoscopy
Peptic ulcer disease		
A break in the lining of the stomach or duodenum.	Abdominal pain Nausea Vomiting Rarely bleeding in the stool	Gastroscopy Blood tests

Table 7.1 Conditions that might be considered before diagnosing coeliac disease *continued*

Condition	*Symptoms	*Tests
Pernicious anaemia		
Auto-immune condition stopping the absorption of vitamin B12.	Tiredness Pins and needles in the feet	Blood tests
Menorrhagia		
Heavy menstruation causing anaemia.	Tiredness, fatigue	Blood tests
Osteoporosis		
Brittle bones.	Bone fracture	Blood tests

*Note: Not all symptoms may be present; and not all tests may need to be ordered.

Treating coeliac disease—a gluten-free diet

The most important treatment for coeliac disease is to remove gluten from the diet. Wheat, barley, rye flour and oats should be immediately taken out of the diet on diagnosis. Unfortunately, this is not as easy as it sounds. Gluten is in many foods that we often don't know about. For example, it is used in many processed foods and sauces such as soy sauce. Wheat flour, which contains gluten, is a cheap, effective thickener and filler in many of the prepared meals on our supermarket shelves, and in many fast foods. It is also used in products like ice cream, pasta, sausages, fish sticks, cheese spreads, salad dressings, soups, sauces, mixed seasonings, mince pies, and some medications and vitamin preparations. You can find it in some brands of instant coffee, tomato sauce, lollies and candy bars, and mustard. These are just a few examples.

Under the Food Standards Code of Food Standards Australia and New Zealand, food manufacturers must list all ingredients on the product packaging. More specifically, there is a mandatory labelling requirement for cereals containing gluten and its products. This requires food manufacturers to list cereals containing gluten, namely, wheat, rye, barley and oats, 'when present in a food as an ingredient, an ingredient of a compound ingredient, a food additive or a processing aid'.

The good news is there are many healthy foods available that do not contain gluten, such as fresh fruit and vegetables, all fresh meats, and staples like maize (corn), potato and rice. See the list below.

Encouragingly, many grocery shops and food outlets now cater for people with coeliac disease by stocking a range of gluten-free foods. Many restaurants and cafes are also becoming aware of the need to provide gluten-free meal options on their menus.

What foods are gluten-free?

In Australia and New Zealand, a **gluten-free** claim can be made if the food contains no detectable gluten and no oats or malt; whereas a **low-gluten** claim can be made if the food contains no more than 20 mg/100 grams gluten and no oats or malt. Food Standards Australia and New Zealand is updating its standards for food labelling, and it is anticipated that when the new labelling takes effect, ALL ingredients known to cause a reaction in sensitive people must be declared on the label—except for labels of beer and spirits.

This means that ingredients that contain gluten, such as starches, thickeners and maltodextrins (a thickening starch), will have to have their source stated on the label, as well as ALL other ingredients in foods (not just cereals) that are known to cause any reaction in sensitive people will also have to be declared on the label—except for beer and spirits. For example, labelling for maltodextrin will have to declare from which gluten-containing grain it was derived. This will also apply to processing aids and compound products, such as the toffee bits in ice cream. Note, however, that ingredients containing gluten-free grains such as corn or maize DO NOT have to be declared on the label.

To help you distinguish foods that contain gluten from those that don't, it is highly recommended that you talk to a dietitian specialising in coeliac disease, and the independent organisation the Coeliac Society of Australia, which has lists of gluten-free products, available to members at www.vic.coeliac.org.au. You may have noticed that there are many free lists on the Internet published by self-help groups—but be wary, as these lists are only useful in the country in which they are compiled because products and laws about food labelling vary.

Generally, if you are on a gluten-free diet, you can eat:

- Fresh fruit and vegetables
- Fresh fish, chicken and red meats—avoid processed meats
- Corn (maize)
- Potato
- Rice and rice flours
- Sago and arrowroot starches
- Soy and soy beans
- Polenta (made with flour)
- Dairy foods—yoghurt, cheese and milk.

What about drugs and alcohol?

The rules are different for drugs. Pharmaceuticals still only have to conform to the International Codex Alimentarious Standard of less than 0.02 per cent gluten to be labelled as 'gluten-free', which is *low gluten* by Australian and New Zealand food standards. Ask your pharmacist before buying medication if it contains trace ingredients that may include gluten.

As for the question of alcohol, all beers, lagers, ales and stouts use gluten products and should be avoided. Alternative alcoholic drinks that are gluten-free include wines, liqueurs and ciders.

Spirits such as brandy and scotch whiskey are okay, but be careful of the double-malted whiskeys.

Gluten-free wheat

A word of caution about gluten-free wheat—while you may be able to find it on the supermarket shelf for home baking, some mills use the same production lines and equipment to process gluten products as they do to process non-gluten products. This can cause contamination and even the tiniest amount of gluten can trigger a reaction in some coeliac sufferers.

Helpful recipe books that publish alternate foods and gluten-free diet plans are available at most good book stores, usually at a reasonable price. You can begin by trying some of the easy-to-follow gluten-free recipes at the end of this book. Some national coeliac associations also provide free recipes; see the resources section at the end of this chapter for more information on these groups.

Tips for living a gluten-free life

- Use separate utensils and working areas when cooking and serving food if catering for people with and without coeliac disease in the same kitchen. Prepare gluten-free food first. Using gluten-free brands can minimise the need to prepare two different meals.
- Clearly label all foods in the refrigerator, freezer and pantry.
- Check food spreads and dips for leftover crumbs that may contain gluten.
- Keep the grill and barbecue clean.
- The toaster is a likely source of contamination with crumbs containing gluten; you may need two toasters.
- Do not get your bread sliced at the bakery as this could cause crumb contamination.
- Don't be afraid to tell friends your dietary needs when invited for dinner—it is better to be honest. Plan ahead—tell

restaurants when you book that you are on a gluten-free diet and may need other menu options.

- When checking labels for sources of gluten, remember to look for hidden sources such as 'modified starch' and 'hydrolysed vegetable protein', which can contain gluten. However, if they are sourced from a gluten-containing grain (i.e. wheat, rye, oats or barley), it will be declared in the ingredients list on the label.
- Join a support group. Not only can it offer useful tips on living with coeliac disease but the group can provide up-to-date food product information. It is also an opportunity to share your thoughts and feelings with people who understand what you are experiencing.

Treating gastrointestinal symptoms

Most of the gastrointestinal symptoms such as abdominal pain, bloating, diarrhoea and constipation should start to gradually subside once you start on a gluten-free diet.

If your symptoms have not subsided, it suggests there is still residual gluten in your diet that has been missed, or there may be another cause other than coeliac disease for the symptoms. In any case, you should go back and see your doctor and dietitian.

Treating deficiencies and complications caused by coeliac disease

For some people, the complications of coeliac disease are more distressing than the gastrointestinal symptoms. Fortunately, these are less commonly seen now that coeliac disease is being detected and diagnosed much earlier than before. Nonetheless, complications of coeliac do arise from time to time: these are listed below.

Anaemia

In more severe cases, coeliac disease can cause iron deficiency anaemia, which is a low red blood cell count. This is because the damaged villi are unable to absorb iron from iron-rich foods like red meat and green leafy vegetables, which is vital to the formation of red blood cells. If you are anaemic, you may feel tired, lethargic, experience shortness of breath, dizziness, have poor memory, or feel the cold. Less commonly, anaemia in coeliac disease can be related to folate and vitamin B12 deficiency.

As well as a gluten-free diet, patients with anaemia may need iron and folate and vitamin B12 supplements. These should be taken on the advice of your doctor and your iron and folate levels should be rechecked after three months of supplement therapy. Iron tablets can cause constipation and an irritable stomach in some people, and therefore should be taken at meal times or on a full stomach. Also, be sure to drink plenty of water to help guard against constipation. Some people also have orange juice with their tablets, as vitamin C improves the body's ability to absorb iron.

Osteopaenic bone disease

Again, in more severe cases of coeliac disease, some patients may not be absorbing enough calcium and develop weak bones, referred to as osteopaenic bone disease. On the advice of your doctor, patients with low calcium levels or X-ray evidence of bone disease are advised to take oral calcium supplements and oral vitamin D, which helps the calcium stay in the bones and is important for bone health. Calcium supplements are best taken separately from meals to improve the absorption of calcium.

Studies have shown that a strict gluten-free diet can protect against further bone loss, and in many cases bone density may improve within a year.

Neurologic symptoms

Rarely, some coeliac sufferers (more likely to be those diagnosed later in life) experience neurologic symptoms such as difficulty maintaining their balance, especially when walking. Usually this is related to vitamin B12 deficiency and is fixed through regular injections every three months. Less commonly, this can be from 'gluten ataxia' and is thought to be caused by gluten-related damage to parts of the brain and spinal cord. Muscle weakness and pins and needles may also occur very occasionally. Not enough studies have been done to understand these symptoms completely, and treatment is difficult. But, in some people, symptoms have improved after taking multivitamins, such as vitamins A, B and E, or calcium. Unfortunately ataxia has not been found to improve with multivitamins or a gluten-free diet.

Fertility problems

Gynaecologic and obstetric problems are more common in women with untreated coeliac disease. About one in three women of child-bearing age with coeliac disease may stop menstruating; this is called amenorrhoea. Women with untreated coeliac disease may have fertility problems or experience miscarriages. Fertility has improved in many women sufferers after starting a gluten-free diet.

Men with untreated coeliac disease can suffer a low sperm count known as azospermia, or impotence. This has been reversed in many cases once a gluten-free diet is started.

Non-diet treatments for coeliac disease

Currently, there are few treatments for coeliac disease other than diet. The exceptions are listed below, but diet remains the key treatment.

Medications

Coeliac disease almost always responds to a gluten-free diet. When this is unsuccessful, the most common reason is that some gluten is sneaking into the diet. If this is not the case, then, in some instances, drug treatment with corticosteroids, such as prednisolone, is needed, along with a gluten-free diet to control the disease. However, very occasionally coeliac disease can be resistant to dietary measures and drug treatment. Occasionally this can be caused by a rare long-term complication of untreated coeliac disease called small bowel lymphoma—a tumour of white blood cells in the small bowel.

Prognosis

People diagnosed with coeliac disease who stick to a gluten-free diet usually have a good recovery and good health outlook with average life expectancy. Generally, the earlier the diagnosis is made, and the sooner the patient starts on a gluten-free diet, the speedier the recovery. Sufferers will begin to feel more energetic and symptoms may start to subside within two weeks. Healing of the villi takes longer and it usually takes more than twelve months to show a full recovery. In some people, it could take up to two years depending on the extent of the damage and the level of compliance with the diet.

Most children who stick to a gluten-free diet return to normal health. In adults, a study of 335 Finnish sufferers found that more than 80 per cent recovered and would enjoy the average lifespan of the population if they strictly complied with the diet.

In more severe cases, some of the less common complications of the disease, such as pins and needles, unsteady walking and weakness of the bones, were not completely reversible.

Some research suggests that coeliac disease is not always a life-long condition. For example, coeliac disease may appear to vanish in children once they reach adolescence. Not a lot is known about why this happens. But the studies suggest that if children diagnosed with coeliac disease do not comply with a gluten-free diet in adolescence and adulthood, often the disease will reappear later in life. The best advice is for children diagnosed with coeliac disease to remain on a gluten-free diet indefinitely.

Follow-up appointments

Traditionally gastroenterologists would do a repeat gastroscopy and small bowel biopsy after twelve months to see that the bowel has healed on the gluten-free diet. Nowadays, some doctors just use blood tests to monitor the response, as the accuracy of the tests has improved markedly in recent years. However, a repeat biopsy twelve months after diagnosis is still recommended.

If you are having problems complying with your diet, go and talk to your dietician. If you need to find a dietitian, ask your doctor, dietitians' association or Australian Coeliac Society. You can find details of these organisations at the end of this chapter. Ask for a dietitian with specialist knowledge of coeliac disease.

Some common questions about coeliac disease

My doctor said I had a negative blood test for coeliac disease but I feel much better on a gluten-free diet. What should I do?

Many people who have irritable bowel syndrome (IBS) also feel better on a gluten-free diet despite not having coeliac disease. This is probably because part of the wheat not absorbed by the body can be fermented by bacteria in the bowel and cause bloating and gas. Another less likely explanation for this is a false negative blood test result. This means the test comes back negative when in fact it is positive. However, modern serology tests for coeliac disease are now approximately 90 to 95 per cent accurate.

> *I am 32 and my husband and I have been trying to have children for several years. My doctor cannot find any physical reason why I can't conceive. My husband was diagnosed with coeliac disease last year—could this be affecting our fertility?*

Yes. Coeliac disease is known to cause amenorrhoea (no periods) in women and azospermia (low sperm count) and impotence in men. Coeliac disease, however, is a rare cause of infertility. It would be worthwhile having your husband's sperm count tested to see if this is the cause of the problem.

> *I have coeliac disease and I feel much better on my gluten-free diet, but I miss drinking beer and want to have a beer with the boys once a week. Surely one or two beers wouldn't hurt?*

Unfortunately most beer contains gluten and would make most people with treated coeliac disease feel quite unwell even after one glass. However, gluten-free beer is available in Australia. Coeliac sufferer and specialist beer brewer John O'Brien makes a gluten-free beer and takes orders online; see his website: www.obrienbrewing. com.au. The Japanese beer 'Sapporo' is very low in gluten and may be an option for some people with very mild disease. An alternative is to have a glass of wine or a mixed drink, as there is no gluten in wine or spirits.

> *My mother-in-law has coeliac disease and uses different cooking utensils for her food at home. When she comes to visit us, do I need to keep her food and utensils separate to ours?*

A lot of people with coeliac disease are so sensitive to gluten that they feel better using a completely different set of utensils for cooking, including toasters, spoons, saucepans, chopping boards, etc. If you have a close relative who visits often, then buying a few extra utensils would give you and your guest peace of mind.

Further information

Medical contacts

Gastroenterological Society of Australia (GESA)
145 Macquarie Street
Sydney NSW 2000
Phone: (02) 9256 5454
Fax: (02) 9241 4586
Email: gesa@gesa.org.au
Website: www.gesa.org.au

American College of Gastroenterology official patient information website: www.acg.gi.org/patients/gihealth/pdf/celiac.pdf.

British charity for people with coeliac disease: www. coeliac.co.uk.

CORE (the working name of the British Digestive Disorders Foundation) website: www.corecharity.org.uk.

Coeliac support groups

The Coeliac Society of Australia
PO Box 703
Chatswood NSW 2057
Phone: (02) 9411 4100
Fax: (02) 9413 1296
www.coeliac.org.au

Australian state branches

Coeliac Society New South Wales
PO Box 703
Chatswood NSW 2057
Phone: (02) 9411 4100
Fax : (02) 9413 1296
Website: www.nswcoeliac.org.au

The Queensland Coeliac Society Inc.
PO Box 2110
Fortitude Valley BC 4006
Phone: (07) 3854 0123
Fax: (07) 3854 0121
Website: http://qld.coeliac.org.au
Email: qld@coeliacsociety.com.au

Coeliac Society of South Australia Inc.
Unit 5, 88 Glynburn Road
Hectorville SA 5073
Phone: (08) 8365 1488
Fax: (08) 8365 1265
Website: http://sa.coeliac.org.au

The Coeliac Society of Tasmania Inc.
PO Box 159
Launceston Tas 7250
Phone: (03) 6427 2844
Fax: (03) 6344 4284
Website: http://tas.coeliac.org.au

The Coeliac Society of Victoria
PO Box 89
Holmesglen Vic 3148
Phone: (03) 9808 5566
Fax: (03) 9808 9922
Email: vic@coeliacsociety.com.au
Website: http://vic.coeliac.org.au

The Coeliac Society of Western Australia
931 Albany Highway
East Victoria Park WA 6101
Phone/Fax: (08) 9470 4122
Website: www.wa.coeliac.org.au

Other coeliac groups
Coeliac Society of New Zealand Inc.
PO Box 35 724
Browns Bay 1330
Auckland
Phone: + 64 (09) 820 5157
Fax: +64 (09) 820 5187
Website: www.colourcards.com/coeliac

American Coeliac Disease Foundation (CDF)
Website: www.coeliac.org

Coeliac UK
Website: www.coeliac.co.uk

Books

Irresistibles for the Irritable and *Two Irresistibles for the Irritable*
Two books by Australian dietitian Sue Shepherd that provide recipes for people needing a gluten-free diet. They also cater for people needing a fructose-free diet or who are lactose intolerant.
   Author: Sue Shepherd
   Publisher: Shepherd Works, 2006
   Available at: www.coeliac.com.au

The Australian Coeliac Handbook
This handbook describes the disease, the diet—with a guide for a healthy daily menu—special facts relevant to children, travelling, dining out, shopping and bread-making, and recipes.
   Author: Australian Coeliac Society
   For details contact your state society: http://coeliac.org.au.

Easy Breadmaking for Special Diets
A handy guide about baking bread for people on special diets. It is ideal for those with bread-making machines.
    Author: Nicolette M. Dumke
    Publisher: Allergy Publications, 1997

Useful websites

GESA has some useful fact sheets about coeliac disease. You can download them at: www.gesa.org.au/consumer/publications/coeliac disease/Coeliac_A4Card.pdf.

The Australian Broadcasting Corporation has a health site with useful information and web links about coeliac disease and other bowel diseases: www.abc.net.au/health/default.htm.

For more information on dermatitis herpetiformis, this British website is useful: www.dermatitisherpetiformis.org.uk.

Dietary information
For recipes and diet plans, see the Australian Coeliac Society website: http://coeliac.org.au/index.htm.

To find an accredited dietitian in your state or territory, go to the Dietitians Association of Australia website. This site also has useful dietary tips and advice: www.daa.asn.au.

For tips on eating healthily and adding fibre to your diet, go to http://www.betterhealth.vic.gov.au.

For vegetarian gluten-free dietary options, see the Vegetarian Society of the United Kingdom website at: www.vegsoc.org/info/gluten.html.

An online information service set up by Australian gastroenterologists and health professionals includes dietary information for coeliac disease and other digestive disorders: www.gastro. net.au.

The Victorian government has initiated a health website with advice relating to a range of conditions including coeliac disease and gluten-free diets: www.betterhealth.vic.gov.au.

8
Inflammatory bowel disease (IBD)

I was diagnosed with Crohn's disease after experiencing abdominal pain on my right side, fevers and diarrhoea for about three months. I was admitted to hospital one night when the pain was unbearable and the doctors thought it was my appendix. It was discovered during the operation that I actually had Crohn's disease. Since then, I have been taking a steroid called prednisolone, and a tablet called mesalazine. My gastroenterologist told me I should stop smoking because it makes Crohn's worse, so I rang Quit and am using patches. That was two months ago, and now I reckon I have more energy than I have had anytime in the past four years. I have even started training for a triathlon. My dad had ulcerative colitis for many years, and eventually had surgery for bowel cancer. Sometimes, I worry that could be me in a few years.

David, 27, electrician

What is inflammatory bowel disease (IBD)?

Inflammatory bowel disease is a term used to describe two bowel diseases that cause inflammation of the small and/or large bowel.

These diseases are Crohn's disease and ulcerative colitis. They are grouped together under the term IBD because their symptoms can be very similar. Both can cause chronic, relapsing inflammation of the bowel and can cause a range of symptoms affecting other parts of the body such as the joints, eyes and skin.

IBD can be a serious problem for sufferers not only because it can be painful but also because it mainly affects the digestive tract. This means that it can interfere with the digestion and absorption of food and the important nutrients, vitamins and minerals that we get from the things we eat.

The abbreviation IBD looks like IBS. They should not be mistaken. IBS refers to irritable bowel syndrome and it is a very different disease to IBD. The key difference is that IBS does not cause physical inflammation of the bowel. Information on IBS is in chapter four. Also, in some countries, like the United Kingdom, IBD is referred to as inflammatory bowel disorders. In Australia, we tend not to use this term, although if you see it written it refers to the same diseases of ulcerative colitis and Crohn's disease.

In this chapter, Crohn's disease and ulcerative colitis will be discussed together for the most part, but where there are important differences, they will be discussed separately.

Crohn's disease

Unlike ulcerative colitis, Crohn's disease can affect any part of the GIT from the mouth to the anus. It was named after the American doctor Burrill Crohn who, along with two colleagues, Leon Ginzburg and Gordon Oppenheimer, described the disease in 1932. It was only for alphabetical reasons that Crohn's name appeared first on their joint presentation paper at a New Orleans medical conference, and as a result the disease they described was named after him. The inflammation of Crohn's disease can affect the full thickness of the bowel, not just the lining of the bowel wall, as is the case with ulcerative colitis. Crohn's disease is more common in the lower part of the small intestine (also known as the terminal ileum) and the large bowel. When it just affects the large bowel, it is called **Crohn's colitis**. If it affects both the small and large bowel, it is called **ileo-colitis**. When just the small intestine is involved, it is called **ileitis**.

Ulcerative colitis

This is inflammation of the lining of the large bowel and rectum. Unlike Crohn's disease, it does not affect the small bowel, oesophagus or any other part of the GIT. When only the rectum is inflamed, this can be called **ulcerative proctitis**. Ulcerative colitis always involves the rectum and a continuous length of large bowel above it; whereas Crohn's disease can affect segments of bowel away from each other, often described as 'skip' lesions.

Who does IBD affect?

It is estimated that about 45 000 Australians have IBD. It affects about two out of every 100 000 Australians. The incidence rate is similar in New Zealand. It is usually diagnosed in people between the ages of fifteen and 30, but it can appear at any age, including in children. There is a second peak of Crohn's disease (particularly Crohn's colitis) that affects older women. More Australians (about 30 000) have Crohn's disease than ulcerative colitis. Researchers have found that IBD is more common in developed Western societies, and the incidence rate is higher in colder climates: in Europe and America, these are places with more northern latitude. IBD affects men and women at about the same rate—slightly more women suffer Crohn's disease and slightly more men are diagnosed with ulcerative colitis.

What causes IBD?

The cause of IBD is unknown. There have been many theories over the years but none has been proven. Some medical scientists think it may be caused by a problem with the body's immune system, or that an infection from bacteria or a virus triggers the immune system to respond in the way that it does, causing the bowel inflammation. We don't know. We do know that IBD is **not** contagious. There is also **no** evidence that diet or stress causes IBD. However, once IBD has been diagnosed, some changes to your diet can help alleviate symptoms. And, once diagnosed, there is no doubt that stress can precipitate a new attack of IBD. There is likely to be a genetic component to IBD, more so in Crohn's disease than ulcerative colitis. The genetic link is complicated and is not fully understood. What is known is that one in five patients diagnosed with IBD will probably have a relative with the disease. Scientists, who are mapping the human genome, have identified several genes that appear to play a role in the inheritance of IBD; the most conspicuous is on chromosome 16 and its exact role in IBD is being studied.

Ethnicity plays a role too. Those of Jewish origin are two to four times more likely to develop IBD than non-Jewish people living in the same area. Jewish people also are more likely to have more than one member of their extended family diagnosed with IBD.

Medical scientists have also considered environmental factors in the study of the causes of IBD. They have found that IBD is less common in people who fit into any or all of these categories: work outdoors, have been breastfed as babies, and are among the *less* wealthy. This is probably because these people have been exposed to their environment from a young age and have developed better immune protection. Breastfed babies are also better protected from some diseases because they get their mother's protection in the milk while they are developing their own immunity.

Smoking is also an interesting factor. In ulcerative colitis, the disease affects more ex-smokers and non-smokers. The opposite is true for Crohn's disease. Smokers are more likely to be diagnosed than non-smokers, and stopping smoking can lead to a huge improvement in the symptoms of the disease.

How do you know you have IBD?

The symptoms of Crohn's disease and ulcerative colitis come and go depending on the amount of inflammation in the bowel. People with IBD can have good weeks and bad weeks. The main symptoms are diarrhoea—sometimes with blood and/or mucus—abdominal pain, weight loss and tiredness.

Diarrhoea

Diarrhoea is a common symptom of IBD, but it does not have to be present. Occasionally some people may complain of constipation, particularly those with distal ulcerative colitis (i.e. the disease is only down near the rectum). But typically the diarrhoea is loose or liquid and may be more common at night. Some people may feel the need to go to the toilet urgently. Once they have been to the toilet, they may feel that they need to go again. Some people may not be able to control the flow and suffer incontinence. Sometimes the diarrhoea is accompanied by large amounts of mucus, often with blood and pus.

Rectal bleeding

Passing fresh blood from the rectum is more typical of ulcerative colitis than Crohn's disease. The blood can pass separately from a bowel action, or it may be mixed up in the stool. Some people with ulcerative colitis might pass blood-stained mucus or bloody diarrhoea. Passing clots is unusual and suggests another cause. About half of Crohn's disease sufferers will not experience rectal bleeding. Bleeding from the rectum is more obvious in ulcerative colitis. In Crohn's disease, bleeding may not be noticeable, but can be detected when a stool sample is tested for blood.

Abdominal pain

Abdominal pain is more frequent and persistent in Crohn's disease than in ulcerative colitis. In Crohn's disease, it can come and go, or be crampy and always present. In ulcerative colitis, pain can vary from a vague discomfort in the lower abdomen, to cramping. Pain is usually worse when the patient is experiencing a severe attack of the disease. The cause of the pain is thought to be increased tension in the bowel when the inflamed bowel wall contracts.

Other symptoms can include loss of appetite (anorexia), nausea, vomiting, fever—when the disease is active—and anaemia (too little iron in the red blood cells). Anaemia can be a consequence of the malabsorption of iron when the bowel is inflamed and of blood loss from the bowel when the disease is active. There may be other signs of malnutrition such as weak bones (osteoporosis), brittle nails and hair breakage. Anaemia in IBD can also be caused by malabsorption of other vitamins (such as vitamin B12) and certain medications (such as salazopyrin and azathioprine).

Non-GIT symptoms

Uncommonly, people who have Crohn's disease or ulcerative colitis also can have symptoms outside the GIT, also called **extra intestinal manifestations**. These can include joint pain, swollen joints or stiffness, particularly of the knees, ankles, elbows and wrists. These often occur at the same time as a bowel flare-up. Also, skin problems, mouth ulcers and eye problems are not uncommon. Skin lesions or rashes can develop as part of IBD but, more commonly, rashes are the result of some of the drugs used to treat IBD. The eyes can also get inflamed; this can cause blurred vision, headache and sensitivity to light (photophobia).

People with IBD are more prone to developing gall stones, kidney stones and other renal and vascular problems. Rarely, the liver can be affected and can cause the skin to turn yellow (jaundice). IBD can also be the cause of blood-clotting problems. These extra symptoms are very rare.

As with any chronic medical condition, people with IBD will need good emotional support. Support groups and further information are listed at the end of this chapter.

Complications of IBD

Although Crohn's disease and ulcerative colitis are very similar, one of the major differences between the two diseases is in their complications. For this reason, their complications are listed separately below.

Crohn's disease

Complications in Crohn's disease can be serious and need to be treated promptly. Unlike ulcerative colitis, rectal bleeding is NOT a complication of Crohn's disease.

Stricture
Stricture is a relatively common complication of Crohn's disease. Healed inflammation from IBD can cause scar tissue to form, which is less flexible than normal tissue. The scar tissue can narrow the bowel (form a stricture) making it more difficult for digested matter to pass through. Some strictures may need to be treated with surgery to widen the bowel and prevent obstruction.

Obstruction

The bowel can become blocked or obstructed by a stricture. This can be life threatening and needs to be treated in hospital. If the bowel is totally obstructed, the surgery must be done immediately.

Fistulas

Fistulas are tunnels or tracts that link one organ to another. Fistulas usually form because of a partial blockage in the bowel, and the body's subsequent effort to find another passage through. Most fistulas are associated with Crohn's disease, probably because of the scarring and stricturing that occurs in the disease. Fistulas can develop a network of passages with many openings that can occur anywhere around the anus, labia, scrotum, buttocks and thighs. Fistulas can also track internally from one part of the GIT to another or to the vagina and parts of the urinary system such as the bladder.

The treatment depends on the location and depth of the fistula. Some heal by themselves. If a fistula becomes blocked, it will get infected and become an abscess. One in four patients with Crohn's disease is likely to have a fistula that develops into an abscess. An abscess is when the tissue around a fistula becomes infected and pus appears. This most often happens in the abdomen and causes the patient to have a fever and a very tender stomach that hurts when touched. This is a serious situation and needs to be treated in hospital with intravenous antibiotics to prevent perforation and peritonitis occurring.

Perforation and peritonitis

This is a life-threatening situation caused by an abscess bursting (or perforating) into the abdominal cavity (the peritoneum). When this happens, the infection (pus) leaks from the abscess into the peritoneum where it can spread to other abdominal organs. The patient will be obviously unwell, and will have a temperature, look pale, and be sweating and unwilling to move because of the pain. Immediate hospital treatment with surgery is needed to flush out the abdominal cavity and remove any damaged tissue. Without surgery, peritonitis can be fatal.

Ulcerative colitis

Complications are less common in ulcerative colitis but perforation can occur in severe disease, usually as a result of a toxic megacolon. Thankfully fistulas are not seen. More common complications of ulcerative colitis are detailed below.

Severe bleeding (haemorrhage)
A severe attack of ulcerative colitis can lead to heavy bleeding of the bowel out of the rectum. The patient will need to go to hospital immediately to have a blood transfusion to replace the lost blood and may need surgery to stop the bleeding. If the bleeding will not stop and blood loss is heavy, the bowel may need to be removed. This is called a **colectomy** and is only done in extreme cases.

Toxic megacolon
Toxic megacolon, also called acute dilatation, is when part of the large bowel (the transverse colon) inflates and gets bigger because of a severe attack of ulcerative colitis. It is life threatening, but rare, occurring in about 5 per cent of severe cases of ulcerative colitis. It is thought to be triggered by too little potassium and a reaction to opiate painkillers. It is treated in hospital, using a drip to give intravenous fluids containing steroids and replacement potassium. If the bowel does not respond to treatment within 24 hours, surgery to remove the bowel needs to be considered to avoid the bowel perforating and causing widespread infection.

Colorectal cancer
A diagnosis of ulcerative colitis slightly increases the risk of developing bowel cancer. The risk is linked to the duration and severity of the disease. It is recommended that after ten years

with ulcerative colitis affecting the whole large bowel, you should have a regular colonoscopy to check for pre-cancerous cells. If none are found, colonoscopies should be repeated every two to three years. Primary Schlerosing Cholangitis, an unusual liver disease sometimes seen along with ulcerative colitis, is associated with a much higher risk of colorectal cancer.

Other considerations

Inflammatory bowel disease generally affects younger people; such as those in their teens, twenties and thirties. The effects of the disease on people in this age group can be very disruptive to their lifestyle, and pose unique problems for younger people which are discussed below.

IBD in children and adolescents

The incidence of IBD is increasing in children. The reasons why are unclear. In children who have not reached puberty, a key feature of the disease is malnutrition, which can present as stunted growth. This could be because of long-standing inadequate nutrition, or treatment of the active disease with drugs such as steroids. Children with IBD need to be encouraged to eat well—make sure they eat foods from the main food groups so that they get enough energy and the vitamins and minerals necessary for growth and development. It is very important that they get enough dietary calcium and may need calcium supplements. Most of our calcium accumulates in our bones during puberty. IBD treatments such as steroids can hamper the movement of calcium into the bones. If your child is not getting enough calcium, they can be at high risk of developing bone disease such as osteopaenia

Some children may need nutritional supplements. Also, children with IBD are at risk of becoming deficient in iron, folate and vitamin B12. Your doctor will check your child's blood for deficiencies. It is also likely they will refer your child to a dietitian with experience in managing IBD in children so that your child's nutritional requirements can be properly monitored and managed.

IBD and fertility, sex and pregnancy

IBD usually affects people during the peak of their reproductive years. The good news is that studies into the effects of the disease on male and female fertility have found that it has minimal impact. Some of the drugs used to treat IBD can reduce male fertility but this is reversed once the medication is stopped.

But, maintaining a sexual relationship when the disease is active and you are suffering bouts of diarrhoea and pain is not easy. IBD can cause sex to be painful in some women. If these are issues that are affecting your relationship, it is important that you talk to your GP. Support groups can also be helpful in discussing these issues.

The effect of pregnancy on IBD is mixed. Generally, for those women who have the active disease at the time of conception, one-third will improve, one-third will worsen and one-third will have unchanged symptoms. For women who do not have the active disease at the time of conception, the rate of relapse is no different to that of non-pregnant women. Once the baby is born the chance of a relapse is small and, if it occurs, it tends to be mild but should be treated quickly to prevent it worsening. Most medications for IBD are safe when used during pregnancy. It is best to check with your doctor if you have concerns but, generally speaking, mothers-to-be with IBD are more likely to give birth to a healthy baby when they continue on their usual IBD medications as opposed to not taking them, as this may trigger a flare-up which is often more stressful to the pregnancy. However, methotrexate is one drug that is dangerous to the developing foetus and should not be taken while you are pregnant, thinking about becoming pregnant or breastfeeding. Most pregnancies carried by women with IBD are normal. The rate of caesarean section is no higher than in the general population.

IBD and oral contraceptives

Research suggests that women who suffer Crohn's disease and take oral contraceptives may have a higher rate of relapse of Crohn's than women who do not take 'the pill'. This is probably because of poor absorption of the contraceptive tablets. To reduce the risk of relapse, pre-menopausal women who need birth control may want to talk to their doctors about methods other than the oral contraceptive for birth control.

How is IBD diagnosed?

IBD is not diagnosed with a simple test. Diagnosis involves your doctor looking at all the signs and symptoms and gathering information through a physical examination, taking a thorough history from you—particularly noting the duration and severity of symptoms—and doing tests including blood, radiographic and endoscopic examinations.

When taking your history, your doctor might also want to know about recent travel, medications you have been on, sexual activity, diet and whether you know of family members who have been diagnosed with IBD. These details could provide information that points to another illness or supports a diagnosis of IBD.

Tests and investigations

Some of the tests and investigations that your doctor may order are described below.

Blood tests

A sample of your blood will be taken, usually from your arm. This blood will be sent to the laboratory to check things such as iron, haemoglobin and other blood components. This will tell the doctor if you are anaemic or malnourished, both of which can be features of IBD. Depending on your symptoms, your doctor may ask the lab to check for other things, such as your hormone levels from your thyroid gland and your calcium levels; and they may do a blood test to rule out coeliac disease.

A stool sample

You may be asked to provide a sample of your stool to be sent to the laboratory to check if you have an infection. The stool can also be tested straightaway for blood by putting it on a reactive stick that changes colour if blood is present.

A colonoscopy (with or without a biopsy)

You will usually need a colonoscopy to see the extent and location of inflammation in the bowel. This will help decide whether you have active disease or not, and whether it is ulcerative colitis or Crohn's disease. A gastroenterologist usually does this examination. It involves using a colonoscope to look inside the bowel. Sometimes biopsies are taken to look more closely at the bowel lining under a microscope. Biopsies are taken with a small instrument that is similar to tweezers. Only very small samples are taken, and the procedure is painless because there are no nerve endings on the lining of the bowel, though sometimes the colonoscopy can be uncomfortable. It can take between five minutes and 30 minutes and is usually done under sedation. See chapter two for more information.

Barium X-ray (meal and enema)

A barium X-ray is often used to determine the extent of the disease. It is particularly good at showing ulcerations, narrowing and fistulas of the bowel. Barium is a chalky material that is visible by X-ray and appears white on X-ray films. There are two types of barium X-ray tests that your doctor might order. One is a small bowel follow-through, also called an upper GI series, which involves drinking the barium so that pictures can be taken of the stomach and the small intestines. The other is a barium enema, which involves administering barium through the rectum via a tube that is inserted into the anus. This allows for pictures to be taken of the large intestine, where ulcerative colitis occurs.

CT scan (computerised axial tomography, also called a CAT scan)

A CT scan is a computerised X-ray that enables imaging of the entire abdomen and pelvis. It is helpful for finding abscesses in the bowel. To prepare for the scan, you might be asked to drink at least two cups of a clear, safe X-ray dye containing iodine to make sharper pictures, and wait an hour to give it a chance to be digested. The test involves lying still on a table while the CT scan moves over you. It can be noisy but no moving parts will touch you. You will be exposed to the same amount of radiation as an X-ray. For this reason the staff will be behind a glass wall while the pictures are being taken, but they will be able to see and hear you. The procedure can take between five and 30 minutes.

MRI (magnetic resonance imaging)

This newly available test provides very clear pictures of the body's organs and tissue by using a magnetic field and radio waves. No X-rays are involved. Remove all metal, jewellery and make-up before the test. Tell your doctor if you are afraid of enclosed spaces or have a pacemaker. The test will take between 30 and 60 minutes, and often you can listen to some music during the examination.

Video capsule endoscopy

This test has recently started to be used as a tool to diagnose Crohn's disease. It involves the patient swallowing a tiny video camera inside a pill the size of a normal capsule. As the capsule journeys through the GIT, it sends video images of the lining of the small intestine to a receiver carried on a belt at the waist. The images are downloaded and then reviewed on a computer. It is an expensive test because the cameras are not reusable. It is also not recommended if it is suspected that the bowel has narrowed because of strictures, as the camera may get stuck and cause an obstruction, or make a pre-existing partial obstruction worse. The value of video capsule endoscopy is that it can identify the early, mild abnormalities of Crohn's disease, which sometimes cannot be picked up by barium X-rays.

Other tests
Most women with abdominal pain will need a gynaecological examination to rule out a gynaecological cause. This normally involves inserting a small plastic speculum into the vagina to allow the doctor to check for any abnormalities.

Distinguishing Crohn's disease from ulcerative colitis

Properly assessing IBD and working out if the diagnosis is Crohn's disease or ulcerative colitis is important, especially when it comes to treatment. For example, ulcerative colitis can be cured by surgery, Crohn's disease cannot.

Sometimes patients will have features of both diseases. When this happens, which is in about 10 per cent of cases, it is called **indeterminate colitis**. If indeterminate colitis is diagnosed, surgical treatments can be less appealing because Crohn's symptoms can develop after surgery.

If it is not IBD, then what?

Table 8.1 Conditions that might be considered before diagnosing IBD

Condition	*Symptoms	*Tests
Coeliac disease		
An intolerance to gluten, a protein found in wheat, barley, rye and oats. Associated with other diseases like Type 1 diabetes. See chapter seven for more detailed information.	Abdominal pain Wind Bloating Diarrhoea and constipation Weight loss Malnutrition Osteoporosis	Blood test Endoscopy
Lactose intolerance		
Unable to absorb lactose, which is found in milk and some dairy products such as yoghurt. Particularly common in people of Asian descent. Caused by a congenital lack of an enzyme, called lactase, that breaks down lactose.	Diarrhoea Wind Abdominal pain Bloating Nausea	Breath test Trial lactose-free diet
Medication side effects		
Unintended and usually unwanted effect of medication.	Abdominal pain Wind Bloating Diarrhoea or constipation Vomiting and nausea Reflux	Blood tests Trial removal of medication or change of medication
Cancer of the colon		
Changes to the cells in the large bowel. Initially there may be few symptoms other than traces of blood in the stool.	Abdominal pain Blood or mucus in stool Weight loss	Colonoscopy Blood test Stool test for blood

Table 8.1 Conditions that might be considered before diagnosing IBD *continued*

Condition	*Symptoms	*Tests
Cancer of the colon continued	Anorexia (lack of appetite) Tiredness Diarrhoea and/or constipation	CT scan
Diverticulitis Inflammation of pockets in the large bowel. Associated with older age and low-fibre diet. For more detailed information, see chapter nine.	Abdominal pain Diarrhoea Fever	Blood tests CT scan Colonoscopy
Tuberculosis (TB) People who develop symptoms overseas, especially in Nepal and South-East Asia, may have a variant of TB which mimics Crohn's disease.	Diarrhoea Rectal bleeding Fever Pain	Colonoscopy Blood test
Irritable bowel syndrome (IBS) A common disorder featuring fluctuating symptoms of abdominal pain and a change of bowel habit.	Abdominal pain Nausea Bloating Diarrhoea and constipation	Gastroscopy Colonoscopy Blood tests
Giardiasis Caused by a parasite that lives in the gut. The source may be untreated water, unwashed foods, unwashed hands, raw meat and pets. Often treated (without a definite diagnosis) with antibiotics.	Abdominal pain Diarrhoea Wind Vomiting and nausea	Stool sample Treatment with antibiotics Endoscopy

Table 8.1 Conditions that might be considered before diagnosing IBD *continued*

Condition	*Symptoms	*Tests
Eating disorders		
A mental illness leading to intentional food deprivation or sporadic consumption of food followed by induced vomiting. The two most common eating disorders are anorexia nervosa and bulimia.	Vomiting Anorexia (lack of appetite) Diarrhoea Constipation Weight fluctuations Tiredness Emotional instability Damaged teeth Reflux Malnutrition Bloating	Psychiatric assessment Blood tests
Microscopic colitis		
Microscopic inflammation of the bowel often associated with certain medications.	Watery diarrhoea that comes and goes	Colonoscopy

*Note: Not all symptoms may be present; and not all tests may need to be ordered.

Treating IBD

The aim of treatment is to put the active disease into remission and to try and prevent a relapse. Treatment options depend on the severity of the disease and what part of the GIT is affected. Drugs play a large role in treating IBD. Surgery is considered in severe cases, and can be a cure for ulcerative colitis. Diet and nutrition also play an important role in managing IBD. Smoking can have a devastating effect on Crohn's disease and should be stopped where appropriate. These treatment options are discussed in more detail below.

First, the severity of the disease needs to be ascertained to determine which drugs will be most suitable with the least amount of side effects. As with many conditions, more powerful drugs for the treatment of IBD often have more serious side effects. Some clinicians define the disease in terms of mild, moderate and severe. This is a modest system, but can be of some use. They are defined as follows:

- Mild—fewer than four stools daily, with or without blood, with no other obvious non-GIT symptoms
- Moderate—more than four stools daily, and there may be minimal non-GIT symptoms
- Severe—more than six stools daily with blood and with other symptoms, including fever, high pulse and anaemia.

Drugs

Generally, if the disease is mild and limited to the left side or rectum, topical therapy may be given in ulcerative colitis. Topical treatments are put directly into the back passage via an enema, foam or suppository (tablet). Topical treatment can also be very effective even in more extensive disease, and is probably under-used in our community.

Most people are treated with oral medications with good effect. Very rarely, IBD sufferers may require admission to hospital for treatment intravenously.

Some of the drug types that may be used by your doctor, depending on the severity and location of the inflammation, are explained below. They may be used in combination, and may be given via a drip in hospital or as a tablet at home, again depending on the severity of the flare-up.

Aminosalicylates (5-ASA compounds)

Drugs belonging to this group include: sulfasalazine, mesalazine and olsalazine.

These drugs are often used in the treatment of ulcerative colitis and in mild to moderate Crohn's disease. They were first used in the treatment of rheumatoid arthritis, and were unintentionally found to have a healing effect on the bowel.

These drugs can induce remission in people with active colitis or proctitis. Once remission is achieved, your doctor may want you to stay on these tablets to maintain the remission. If a flare-up recurs, increasing the dose for a short time can sometimes best treat this.

Antibiotics

Drugs belonging to this group include: metronidazole (Flagyl), ciprofloxacin, clarithromycin, rifampicin, ethambutol, dapsone, clofazimine and vancomycin.

Antibiotics play an important role in treating Crohn's disease and the complications of Crohn's disease such as fistulas. One theory of the cause of Crohn's disease is that it results from the overgrowth of intestinal bacteria. Antibiotics attack bad bacteria (and unfortunately good bacteria too!). One bacterium that has been singled out is a type of bacterium similar to the micro-organism responsible for tuberculosis. This intestinal bacterium is called *Mycobacterium avium* subspecies *paratuberculosis* (MAP). If this theory were correct, it would explain why antibiotics could be effective in the treatment of Crohn's disease, particularly Crohn's colitis. More research needs to be done on this subject before we will know conclusively.

However, antibiotics are not the key to the treatment of ulcerative colitis. Generally, it is thought that antibiotics are unnecessary in the treatment of ulcerative colitis unless there is another reason for using them, such as infection or abscess.

Glucocorticoids (steroids)

Drugs belonging to this group include: prednisolone, hydrocortisone acetate and budesonide.

Steroids are often the first choice of treatment because they work very quickly and can be given by tablet or topically via the back passage in the form of an enema or foam injection.

Steroids are also good for treating flare-ups as well as helping non-GIT symptoms such as painful joints and skin and eye problems. They can be given orally or through a drip depending on the severity of the flare-up. Steroids are not recommended for maintaining disease remission because they do not prevent relapse and they have quite a few side effects when used long-term.

In high doses and when used long-term, the unpleasant side effects of steroids that you need to be aware of include: increased appetite and weight gain, 'moon' face, acne, increased facial hair, high blood sugar level and propensity to develop diabetes, increased blood pressure, mood swings, insomnia, and tendency to bruise more easily; long-term use can also weaken bones (osteoporosis). Your doctor will weigh up the side effects with the benefits, and discuss them with you, if you need steroids long-term.

Steroids should NOT be stopped abruptly—this could upset your natural hormone levels and make you very sick. The steroid dose needs to be gradually reduced and your doctor will advise you how to do this. If you take steroids regularly and miss doses because of illness or vomiting, you need to contact your doctor immediately.

Immunosuppressive agents
Drugs belonging to this group include: cyclosporine, methotrexate and thiopurine agents. Thiopurine agents include: Azathioprine (Imuran), and 6-mercaptopurine (6-MP, Puri-Nethol).

These drugs are used to treat active disease and to maintain remission in people who have not responded to other types of treatment such as steroids, antibiotics and 5-ASAs. Cyclosporin is usually reserved for people with severe ulcerative colitis at risk of immediate perforation or megacolon. Thiopurine agents have been found in studies to be good at healing fistulas, which are common in Crohn's disease.

Unfortunately it can take a few months before these drugs achieve their maximum benefit. Your doctor may start you on these before stopping other medications, to allow for the lag time until the drug is effective. Immunosuppressive agents should not be given as a first treatment option. These drugs are very safe, but rarely can cause serious side effects that you need to know about. As the name suggests, these drugs suppress the immune system which can be a good thing for slowing down IBD, but long-term use can affect the bone marrow where red and white blood cells are made, making it difficult for the body to fight other infections. There is also a very slight increase in the risk of developing cancer such as lymphoma—this risk is only very slight, but you should be aware of it. For this reason, monthly blood tests are recommended while using these drugs, to check the health of the bone marrow. Crohn's disease itself probably also slightly increases the risk of developing lymphoma.

Methotrexate is another drug that was best known for treating skin conditions such as psoriasis and the debilitating joint disease, rheumatoid arthritis. It was in the treatment of these illnesses that the drug was found to be of use in bringing about remission in people with quite severe IBD. It is not a drug that should be taken without due consideration. Side effects can include: nausea, diarrhoea, hair loss, and low white cell levels in the blood. It is also thought to cause liver and lung problems in some people, which can be irreversible. Moreover, methotrexate is dangerous to unborn babies and should never be given to pregnant or breast-feeding women. Women taking methotrexate should always have a reliable method of contraception.

Infliximab

Infliximab is a new and exciting treatment, used mainly for Crohn's disease, that has been designed by scientists to attack one of the chemicals that causes inflammation in the bowel. Inflix-imab is a chemical that neutralises Tumour Necrosis Factor (TNF) and is comprised of proteins derived from both humans and mice. Because of this, it is very expensive to produce, and can occasionally cause allergic reactions. It is given intravenously over a couple of hours and possibly repeated after a few weeks as necessary. It has been very successful for treating Crohn's disease that has not responded to all other treatment, and works in approximately 70 per cent of these patients. It also can have a miraculous effect on fistulising disease. Despite Infliximab's success in treating Crohn's disease, the Australian government currently does not provide this drug on the PBS for Crohn's disease, but does for rheumatoid arthritis. Because of this, Infliximab is generally only available through public hospitals at present. A campaign urging the Australian federal government to reconsider this decision is underway by various support groups such as the Australian Crohn's and Colitis Association.

Other treatments

Anaemia

This is a common problem in IBD and often overlooked—even by gastroenterologists. Anaemia is often a result of iron deficiency related to poor absorption and bleeding, but also can be due to causes such as vitamin B12 deficiency (Crohn's disease) and from the disease itself. Iron tablets are sometimes poorly tolerated in IBD and might even make inflammation worse. In this situation, iron is often given intravenously with good effect. Very rarely IBD patients may also need a blood transfusion.

Replacement fluids and electrolytes

Replacement fluids and electrolytes are often needed if IBD is severe and requires hospitalisation. This is done by putting a drip into the arm.

Total parenteral nutrition (TPN)

In severe cases of IBD, where the GIT has been unable to absorb necessary nutrients for some time, TPN, or intravenous nutrition, may be given through a drip inserted into a major vein. The catheter that goes into the vein is called a central venous catheter (CVC). Giving nutrition through a CVC allows the GIT time to rest and heal. It is very important to keep the CVC site very clean to prevent an infection getting into the body. TPN contains all the essential vitamins, minerals and nutrients that the body needs. TPN should not be used unless completely necessary, because of complications such as infection, and shrinkage of the bowel lining. For this reason, your doctor will want to get the GIT functioning as soon as possible by starting you on fluids as soon as you are up to it.

Nutrition and IBD

So far, there has been no scientific evidence that a specific diet can prevent disease flare-ups in adults. There is no special diet for IBD, therefore be cautious of any diet that claims to be 'the IBD diet'. This is not to say that nutrition is not important. On the contrary, it is paramount for all IBD sufferers to pay close attention to their diets to make sure they are getting the nutrients they need, and to maintain a healthy weight.

The role of nutrition as a therapy is based on improving and maintaining good nutritional status. A small number of patients may need to modify their eating patterns to maintain their body weight, correct nutritional deficiencies and alleviate symptoms of IBD. In children, diets may be modified to promote growth and development. Thus, the adjustments made to your diet will depend on the severity of your disease, nutritional requirements, weight and personal taste.

Healthy adults need to consume between 6800 kJ (1700 Cal) and 9200 kJ (2300 Cal) a day, depending on their height and body weight. People with IBD and who are underweight generally need an extra 10 to 20 per cent added to their caloric intake to improve their health. It is also thought that people with IBD need more daily protein (about 1.2 grams per kilogram of body weight). High-energy, protein drinks can help meet these targets. Foods that are high in protein include red meat, fish, chicken, eggs, tofu, milk and dairy products.

Nutritional needs will be different for people with ulcerative colitis compared to Crohn's disease. Crohn's can affect the whole digestive tract from the mouth to the anus, whereas ulcerative colitis affects the colon only. This means that these diseases have different impacts on a patient's nutritional status.

Chapter one explained the role of the GIT in the digestion of nutrients, minerals and vitamins and their absorption. Most nutrients are absorbed in the small intestine. In ulcerative colitis, inflammation occurs only in the large bowel and rectum; and, as most nutrients have been absorbed into the body by this stage in the digestion process, ulcerative colitis, compared to Crohn's disease, is less frequently associated with deficiencies and malnutrition. The frequencies of nutritional disorders that occur in IBD patients are shown in Table 8.2 (see page 200).

Dietary considerations during a flare-up of IBD

Nutritional requirements during an attack, usually of Crohn's disease, are based on identifying nutrient deficiencies and correcting them. These problems need to be treated to prevent the immune system becoming weaker and leaving the patient susceptible to further flare-ups and delays in healing. If surgery has been done in the past, or there have been multiple bowel resections, some people can develop a condition called **short bowel syndrome**. This means that they are unable to properly absorb enough nutrients in the remaining bowel to maintain good health. In some very rare cases, people with short bowel syndrome may need life-long TPN. But, to reiterate, this is very rare and should not cause undue concern.

Depending on the severity of the inflammation—and again, this information is for a small minority of IBD patients with severe inflammation who have been hospitalised—nutrients can be given enterally, this means into the stomach, again in liquid form, through a nasogastric tube or, if the patient is well enough, via the mouth. Enteral feeding is sometimes called tube feeding because it often involves inserting a nasogastric tube into the nose, down the gullet and into the stomach.

Table 8.2 Nutritional disorders that can occur in IBD

Nutritional disorder	Crohn's disease %	Ulcerative colitis %
Underweight	70	18–55
Lactose intolerance	30–40	25–65
Protein deficiency (hypoalbuminemia)	25–80	0–10
Anaemia	25–85	22–68
Low folic acid	50–79	5–20
Low vitamin B12	16–39	8–30
Low iron	10–44	30–80
Bone weaknesses (osteopathies)	24–39	0–15
Calcium deficiency	20–60	0–46
Magnesium deficiency	30–68	2–55
Zinc deficiency	42–92	12–52

Source: Falk Foundation

Enteral diets

An enteral diet can also be referred to as a fluid diet, elemental diet or astronaut diet. The latter term arose because the American space centre, NASA, first developed these liquid foods for its astronauts. The idea was to make a food that was high in energy, protein and essential vitamins and minerals but without roughage so that all the food could be absorbed without the body needing to produce faeces. This meant food was smaller and astronauts wouldn't have to store the extra weight of faecal waste in the spacecraft for disposal back home. Interestingly, the diet was never used the way it was intended because it was said that the astronauts found it unpalatable. This was probably because proteins that are broken down into amino acids can have an offensive smell. But doctors realised the benefits of this efficient, high-energy diet for IBD sufferers because the absence of fibre meant less work for the bowel, thereby allowing it time to rest and recover.

The specially prepared enteral and parenteral diets for IBD and some short bowel syndrome patients have all the high energy, protein and vital nutrient and active substances to provide nutrition and help the body heal. Some of these diets are high molecular weight fluid diets (also called nutrient-defined diets or polymeric diets), and some are low molecular weight diets (also called chemically defined diets or elemental diets). The central difference is that the low molecular weight diets have already had the major nutrients (fat, protein and carbohydrate) broken down into more easily absorbed molecules. Studies have been done to see if these specially prepared high and low molecule diets improve healing times—but the results are mixed. The theory behind enteral and parenteral diets is that they may inhibit GIT immune responses and reduce inflammation. They may also encourage healing of the bowel wall and reduce the amount of bad bacteria in the small bowel. To date, there is no conclusive evidence that enteral and parenteral diets actually bring about remission in adults suffering an IBD flare-up. Also, scientific studies have found that low molecular weight diets are no better than high molecular weight diets in improving the health of IBD patients.

However, the results were promising in children. Enteral nutrition is especially used in children with IBD to prevent malnutrition and to encourage growth. It has been found to be as effective as steroids in inducing remission in some children. In adults, this is not the case. This is not to say that these diets do not have a role: they are useful in improving the nutritional status of people with severe IBD.

What to eat after a flare-up

Your dietitian will look at your individual needs and recommend what type of diet suits you best. Regular blood tests may be necessary to check your levels of essential vitamins and minerals, especially calcium and zinc: if your levels are low, you may need a supplement until your levels improve. Many of these are available in tablet form without prescription; that is, 'over the counter'. But do not be tempted to self-diagnose. Most people with IBD do not require vitamin and mineral supplements. If you are taking supplements you don't need, it can be a waste of money and most are excreted in the urine because the body is unable to store them.

Most dietitians recommend that patients with IBD eat whatever they can tolerate. The best way to get nutrients, vitamins and minerals is in food. But keep a food diary so that you can see which foods disagree with you and which nutrients you may be missing out on. Foods that are often hardest to tolerate are: fatty foods, acidic foods, milk, onions, citrus fruits, fruit juice, raw vegetables and legumes. Some people may have other, co-existing intolerances such as lactose intolerance and fructose intolerance, which might be contributing to their symptoms.

But, no one can tell you which foods you will not tolerate, because everyone is different. Lists of foods that are hard to

Food	Time	Complaint/commentary

handle for people with IBD can be unhelpful because they can create fear of those foods. You need to find out for yourself by keeping a food diary. It might look something like this.

In the complaints column, make sure you note if you experienced pain or bloating, or if there was a bowel movement and what it was like: watery, soft, thin, etc. You will soon identify foods you cannot tolerate. Avoid these for the time being (short-term). When you feel well again, try them again. It is very important to remember that intolerances can resolve themselves.

Start with foods that are generally better tolerated. These often include: fish, cooked meat, chicken, rice, pasta, cooked fruit, and cooked vegetables. Add bread, butter, jam, lunch meat and cheese to give you more dietary options if you think you can tolerate it. Add a new food every two or three days and see how it makes you feel. You should also keep an eye on your weight—measure it every week on the bathroom scales to make sure it is not too low for your height. See your doctor if your weight starts to drop.

Lactose intolerance

People with inflammation in the small intestine caused by Crohn's disease may develop a temporary intolerance to the sugar in milk called **lactose**. This is because the inflammation may reduce the amount of the enzyme, called lactase, that breaks down lactose. Lactase is produced in the small bowel lining.

If lactose is not being broken down properly into its smaller sugar parts, more than usual amounts of lactose will reach the large bowel. Lactose attracts water into the large bowel, meaning that less water than normal is absorbed back into the body. Also, the normal bacteria in the large bowel use lactose and this process causes by-products to form that speed up the motility of the bowel wall (peristalsis), and it also causes gas. Together, the increased water and increased motility cause more diarrhoea. Lactose intolerance is usually temporary and will resolve a few weeks after the inflammation has settled down. In the meantime, avoid large amounts of milk, yoghurt and ice cream. Soft cheeses contain small amounts of lactose; choose lactose-free varieties if available. Interestingly, hard cheese is lactose free and is generally okay. Soy milk or rice milk (with calcium added) are good supplements to use instead of cow's milk because they do not contain lactose.

Beverages

People with IBD need to keep their fluids up. Healthy adults need a minimum of 1.5 litres a day of fluid to keep their body functioning well. People with IBD may lose a lot of fluid through diarrhoea and will need much more than this to compensate for the loss. Your doctor or dietitian will be able to advise you on how much you will need depending on the severity of your disease. As a general rule, try and drink at least eight glasses of water each day. Avoid any drinks that cause symptoms (e.g. fruit juices). Also, if you have Crohn's disease, you may need to avoid milk drinks during a flare-up because you may be lactose intolerant temporarily.

The role of prebiotics, probiotics and more

Prebiotics

Prebiotics promote the growth of good bacteria in the gut. Usually they consist of carbohydrates that cannot be digested by the body. In other words, they are a type of dietary fibre. They are being studied for their role in supporting good bacteria in the GIT. Micro-organisms in the GIT are also called **intestinal flora**. Some of these micro-organisms are good and help us break down food ready for absorption, while others are bad and cause infection. Prebiotics are food for the good intestinal flora. Examples of foods containing prebiotics include garlic, asparagus, onions, yoghurt and milk.

Probiotics

Probiotics are living micro-organisms. Probiotic means 'for life'. They are so-called good bacteria—including certain strains of lactobacilli, found in some yoghurt cultures—that can help the GIT fight against infection from bad bacteria, viruses and fungi. They exist naturally in your intestine. Your levels of 'good bacteria' can fall sharply if you are taking antibiotics. This is because antibiotics are unable to discriminate between good and bad bacteria and wipe out both. This can cause problems such as diarrhoea, pain, nausea and bloating.

Probiotics are thought to work by attaching to the intestinal wall of the bowel and stopping the bad pathogens getting through. They keep the bad bacteria under control. It is also thought that they help temporary lactose intolerance because some probiotic bacterial strains produce bacterial lactase and can help the body digest the milk sugar called lactose. In order to take advantage of the good work of probiotics, you need to have one or two servings of probiotic-enriched food a day.

Probiotics have become somewhat of a buzz word in digestive health over the past decade in the Western world, and are being studied at major research hospitals to evaluate their usefulness in the treatment of IBD, diarrhoea, and fungal infections such as thrush, and to counter the negative effects of antibiotics. Eastern countries such as Japan have been using probiotics for years to improve digestion and maintain good health. There is good evidence that probiotics can help prevent developing travellers' diarrhoea and they are used by the US army for this reason.

Food marketers have jumped on the probiotic bandwagon by promoting products that contain probiotics. Most probiotics taken by mouth do not survive the acidic environment in the stomach, and a large number of probiotic preparations available in pharmacies are often dead when sold. Many probiotics require refrigeration. Speak to your doctor or pharmacist about which suit your needs. Examples of probiotics available in supermarkets and pharmacies include Yakult, USL3 and Inner Health Plus.

Synbiotics

A synbiotic is a food product that contains both prebiotics and probiotics. It is thought that synbiotics improve the survival of the probiotic organism by providing the material the probiotic organism needs.

Fish oil capsules

Another fashionable complementary treatment for IBD is fish oil, either fresh, or via a capsule from your pharmacist. Fish oil contains the active ingredient eicosapentaenoic acid. Fish oil is also sometimes recommended for lowering the risk of heart disease and stroke. This is because a component of fish oil, omega-3, has been proven to reduce cholesterol in the bloodstream. Eicosapentaenoic acid is a special component of fish fat that is thought to prevent inflammation by blocking the release of bad substances that cause it. So far, studies have shown that fish oil works better for people with ulcerative colitis than Crohn's disease. One problem with fish oil is that you need a lot of it to get a response. More research needs to be done into the effects of fish oil on inflammation before it can be recommended as a remedy. These days surgery is not commonly required for IBD. However, though less often, in selected cases it is still the best option and can improve a patient's quality of life. Surgery options are discussed here.

Surgery and IBD

Ulcerative colitis

The removal of the large bowel can effectively cure ulcerative colitis. But this is major surgery and should not be considered as a first option. If surgery is done electively in ulcerative colitis, generally the large bowel and rectum are removed, and a pouch or reservoir is made from the small bowel, sometimes in two stages, to take the place of the colon as a 'holding area' for faeces. This can be a life-changing operation and even if the pouch is working correctly, patients often still have four to five bowel actions per day. Surgery can also occasionally reduce fertility and male sexual function (about 10 per cent of cases), which obviously should be discussed with your doctor beforehand. Complications of surgery include infection, incontinence, and pouchitis, an inflammation of the pouch that responds very well to probiotics.

In an emergency scenario, generally the large bowel is removed, with a very small rectal stump left behind, and the small bowel is connected to the abdominal wall via a stoma that is then connected with a pouch at a later date. A stoma, or ostomy, is the opening that allows faecal material to leave the body. It is more fully described in chapter eleven.

Four reasons why your doctor may recommend you have surgery are:

- Severe attacks that fail to respond to medical therapy
- Complications of a severe attack (e.g. perforation, acute dilatation)
- Chronic ongoing disease that severely restricts your quality of life
- Development of pre-cancerous cells or cancer.

Crohn's disease

Surgery in Crohn's disease is used to control symptoms and treat complications. With the advent of new medications, surgery is now used rarely in treating Crohn's disease. Older studies have found that the more time that passes since diagnosis, the greater the likelihood of needing surgery. Between 25 and 45 per cent of patients have some type of bowel surgery three years after diagnosis. Recurrent surgery is more likely once surgical intervention has occurred. For this reason, if surgery is needed, the goal is to keep as much of the functioning bowel as possible. The main reasons for surgery are fistulas, abscess, haemorrhage, perforation, cancer, toxic megacolon, strictures and bowel obstruction. Surgery is considered in children who are failing to grow.

Surgery does not cure Crohn's disease. The main types of surgery commonly performed are:

- Partial bowel resection
- Strictureplasty
- Correction of fistulas
- Draining of an abscess.

Partial bowel resection

This is done when a portion of bowel is so damaged by the disease that a permanent partial obstruction occurs. The most common sites where this happens are the terminal ileum, the ileo-caecal valve, and the large intestine. If possible, the most straightforward procedure is to cut out the diseased part of the bowel and **anastomose** (join) the healthy ends. This is not always possible and sometimes a temporary opening (ostomy) will need to be created through the abdominal wall with a bag attachment to collect the faecal matter while the bowel is given time to rest before being anastomosed.

Sometimes, after surgery, the disease can flare up above the surgical point, probably because of stricturing occurring at the old anastomosis site. Studies have found that the longer the stretch of time between diagnosis and first surgery, the longer the period between first and second surgery, if it is needed. Some of the 5-ASA drugs have been found to delay post-surgery flare-ups.

Strictureplasty

As the name suggests, this is surgery to open up a narrowing of the bowel caused by scar tissue. A cut is made along the stricture to widen the area. It is then re-sewn.

Correcting fistulas

A fistula is an unintended tunnel between one organ and another. In IBD, fistulas generally occur after a long-standing obstruction, where the bowel tries to make a new passage, often into another area of bowel, or the skin. Fistulas are now often treated with

Infliximab, but sometimes the fistula can be completely removed surgically. Perianal fistulas (occurring near the anus) are usually treated with a Seton procedure. This involves placing a soft silk suture in a loop through the fistula. This doesn't get rid of the fistula, but prevents the fistula becoming blocked and infected. Often this is done as a short-term measure while waiting for other medical treatment (such as azathioprine or Infliximab) to work.

Draining abscesses

If antibiotics are unable to resolve an abscess, it must be drained so that the bowel can heal. The most common method is to insert a hollow needle through the skin into the bowel to reach the abscess and drain it. In more extreme cases, a surgeon may need to open up the area to drain the pus and wash the surrounding tissue.

Preparing for surgery

If you do need to have surgery, here are some practical things you can do to prepare yourself physically and emotionally for the operation:

* Get as much information as you can so that you know what to expect during your recovery. Talk to your gastroenterologist about your treatment options after surgery to prevent a recurrence. It might also be worth talking to a colitis support group or someone who has experienced surgery so that you can be better prepared.
* Look after yourself. Try and improve your nutrition and weight before surgery so that your body is less stressed and better able to heal during the recovery phase.
* Put plans in place so that you are not under undue stress during recovery. Talk to the hospital about getting some help with housework. Organise friends and family to take over chores for a few weeks.

- Talk to your employer. Be as honest as you can to help them to understand that you will need to take sick leave for several weeks while you recover. You don't want to be receiving work calls a few days after surgery.
- Prepare the house. If you live in a house with stairs, consider moving furniture temporarily so that you can live downstairs while you are getting better. Stock up the refrigerator with soft, low-residue foods recommended by your dietitian. Pay bills in advance if you can afford it so that you don't have to worry after surgery.

Recovery from surgery

Don't be alarmed if the initial bowel actions after surgery are liquid. If the large bowel has been removed (colectomy), the small bowel will adapt and will slowly take over some of its functions. Bowel actions will become firmer as the body adapts to the changes and the small bowel starts to absorb more water.

Depending on the type of surgery you have had, you may need supplements. If a large amount of the ileum is removed, you may need vitamin B12 injections every three months as a supplement. You may also need a tablet called cholestyramine (Questran) to help the bowel absorb bile salts, as the failure to absorb these salts can cause fatty diarrhoea (steatorrhoea).

Other post-surgery tips include:

- Follow medical and nursing advice. Get out of bed while in hospital. Do the exercises recommended by the physiotherapist. Keep up to date with pain relief medications. You may feel fine now, but in a few hours you won't if you forget to take your tablets. The sooner you are up and moving, the lower the risk of complications soon after surgery. Movement will also help to get your bowel functioning so that you can begin to try a liquid diet and then low-residue food.
- Once you start drinking, keep up your fluids. This helps the body to remove waste and will make you feel better.

- Limit visitor numbers and allocate rest time. You have had bowel surgery and need to give your body time to heal. Seeing visitors is cheering, but it can also be tiring. Your friends will understand.

- Stick to the rules: no heavy lifting, no driving for a few weeks, and no sex. Your muscles and tissue need time to heal. Your doctor will want to see you for a check-up several weeks after discharge from hospital; then you can ask them when you can start to resume some of these activities.

- Don't be afraid to ask questions. You are going home with a stoma—so make sure you feel confident about managing it before you leave hospital. It is easier to get help when you are in hospital supported by nurses and the in-house stoma therapist.

Prognosis

More is becoming known about the long-term outlook for people with IBD. The good news is that most people can be well controlled on regular medications and go on to live a normal life. Not smoking definitely improves the long-term outcome with Crohn's disease. Genetic testing will become clinically available in the next few years, and this will further help people to predict what they have to expect in the future. The exact course for a person with Crohn's disease is difficult to predict, especially now that new treatments have significantly improved the long-term outlook in Crohn's disease. Disease in the large bowel is often more easily treated than in the small bowel, and once a person requires one operation for Crohn's, their chances of needing further surgery are increased.

Most people with ulcerative colitis have only intermittent attacks of disease, with periods of remission in between that can last for months to years. After the first year from diagnosis, surgery is rarely required in ulcerative colitis. Each year about 1 per cent of people with ulcerative colitis need their bowel removed. People with disease that only affects the end of the large bowel generally fare better, and most of these people only ever have disease at the end of their bowel. There is an increased risk of bowel cancer in those with ulcerative colitis, particularly after ten years of disease. Because of this, it is recommended that these people have regular colonoscopies for cancer surveillance after ten years of disease. Cancer is more common in people with pancolitis—disease throughout the large bowel—and the risk may be reduced in those on aminosalicylate medications.

Coping with a chronic IBD

Crohn's disease and ulcerative colitis are difficult diseases to cope with because they affect all aspects of life. The unpredictability of the illnesses makes it difficult to plan life's daily activities, whether it is the grocery shopping or a social function; in the back of your mind, you are always wondering where the closest toilet is. IBD is an illness that affects people in their prime of life, and this can affect body image and intimacy. It is difficult to feel desirable and be sexually active when your bowels have other urgent plans. Travel may also be difficult because of the fear that you may experience a flare-up or be caught short with no toilet nearby. IBD can cause absences from work and study, which can make professional advancement difficult. Together, these factors can leave you feeling depressed and frustrated. Coping with a chronic illness is not easy. But there are some things you can do to get a bit more control back in your life.

Learn to be a planner

You don't have to stop doing things because you have IBD, but you do need to become a good planner to manage your illness.

Be prepared. When you are going out for the day, pack a small bag with things you could need in an emergency. Be practical. Make a mental note of where the toilets are when you arrive. Carry extra underwear and toilet paper so that you don't get caught if public toilets are not well equipped. Take your medications with you in case you get an attack of pain. If you are ordering food, choose things that you know are the least likely to disagree with you. If possible, telephone ahead to see if there are menu options that suit you.

If you are going on a longer outing or a holiday, plan an itinerary with frequent toilet breaks. Don't try to do too much in one day. Enjoy the slower pace of life, which is what holidays are all about. In case of emergencies, take extra prescriptions with you should you need medication in a hurry. Also, take a letter explaining your condition with your doctor's details, including phone numbers, and medication needs. Make sure your health insurance or Medicare details are with you and up to date. If you are travelling further a field, let your doctor know beforehand and follow their advice.

Get the support you need

Part of dealing with a problem is having someone to share it with. You need to seek out people that you trust and who can support you. This could be your local doctor, a support group or a bunch of friends who know you well and are understanding. Be as honest with your friends as you can. Let them know your needs so that these can be factored into the day. If you are not feeling well and have to cancel a social occasion, tell them why. Good friends do understand. The same advice goes for partners and employers. Most people appreciate honesty.

People with IBD know the value of sharing their feelings and most cities have a support group. See the end of this chapter for details. Don't feel daunted about joining a group: You can be as involved as much or as little as you want to be. Just reading the group's regular newsletter may be enough for you to feel that you are not alone and to pick up some useful hints about how other people manage their illness.

Don't let fear dictate decisions

It is understandable to be worried about life's choices when you have a chronic illness. But don't let it stop you from trying new things. You still need to be realistic in your employment decisions and other choices by not taking on a commitment that will be difficult to fulfil. You should know your own limits. A high-pressure job with lots of overseas travel may not suit you if you know that you are sick for several weeks a year. That said, allow yourself to experience the things other people your age do. It's okay that sometimes events won't go according to plan. This happens to everyone. The important thing is that you were prepared to give it a go. More often than not, it may work out better than you had hoped.

Some common questions about IBD

Will I always have to take medication for my IBD?

No. Sometimes people are advised to keep taking their medications even if they have been well for some time, but generally medications are not required if you have been in remission for two years.

I want to change jobs, but am worried about telling a new employer that I have IBD. What should I do?

Don't feel you have to tell them anything. Your medical condition is your business and should not be a reason to hold you back from employment. You have a right to expect adequate facilities such as access to toilets and opportunity to take medications if necessary.

If I am stressed, my IBD flares up. Is there a link?

Yes. Stress is a common precipitant for IBD flare-ups. The scientific reason for this is not known but there is no doubt that stress can cause attacks of the disease.

I have read about special diets that can prevent flare-ups. Do these really work?

No. There is some case for special diets for children in IBD but for most people it is important to maintain a good balanced diet with lots of protein. It may be appropriate to avoid fibre if you have stricturing disease, and sometimes lactose during an acute flare-up.

My husband wants to go overseas on holiday for three weeks at the end of the year; I am worried about travelling with IBD. What should I do?

You should discuss this with your doctor. Generally, travel is no problem; however, it might be worth taking a supply of medication, such as prednisolone or some antibiotics, in case you get into trouble. If you do take medication with you overseas, remember to take a letter from your doctor to explain why you need it.

Are there any alternative therapies that I can try to stop the flare-ups?

Sure, there are lots of therapies available on the Internet—but most of them are not supported by scientific evidence and are probably best avoided. Other less conventional therapies available include fish oil (an anti-oxidant) and probiotics. Generally, these are safe to use but are best discussed with your doctor first. Avoiding stress is also important and some alternative therapies discussed in chapter ten can help you learn to relax.

> *I am 28 and have just found out that I am pregnant with my first child; I have had a miscarriage in the past. Should I keep taking my IBD medications during pregnancy?*

Most medications are very safe when used during pregnancy. In general, mothers with IBD are more likely to give birth to a healthy baby when they continue on their usual medications as opposed to stopping everything, as this generally leads to a flare-up which is often more dangerous to the pregnancy. It is always a good idea to discuss pregnancy (both before and during) with your doctor when possible.

> *My wife was diagnosed with ulcerative colitis at 21. What is the likelihood my children will get IBD?*

There is a slightly increased risk of IBD in first-degree relatives of people with IBD (lifetime risk 10 per cent). Having said that, the vast majority of people with relatives with IBD have no trouble.

> *Can exercise help control my IBD?*

Anything that reduces your stress is likely to reduce the risk of having a flare-up in the future. Also, exercise in general obviously makes you healthier and should be recommended in moderation.

Further information

Medical contacts

Gastroenterological Society of Australia (GESA)
145 Macquarie Street
Sydney NSW 2000
Phone: (02) 9256 5454
Fax: (02) 9241 4586
Email: gesa@gesa.org.au
Website: www.gesa.org.au

British Society of Gastroenterology
3 St Andrews Place
Regents Park
London NW1 4LB
Phone: +44 (0) 20 7935 3150
Fax: +44 (0) 20 7487 3734
Email: bsg@mailbox.ulcc.ac.uk
Website: www.bsg.org.uk

American College of Gastroenterology official patient information website: www.acg.gi.org/patients/patientinfo/ibd.asp.

IBD support groups

Australian Crohn's and Colitis Association (ACCA)
Level 1, 462 Burwood Road
Hawthorn, Vic. 3122
Phone: (03) 9815 1266
Website: www.acca.net.au
Email: info@acca.net.au

Or, contact the ACCA office in your state:

New South Wales	Phone: 1800 220 522
Northern Territory	Phone: 1800 220 522
Queensland	Phone: 1800 220 522
South Australia	Phone: (08) 8449 4357
Tasmania	Phone: (03) 6437 6184
Victoria	Phone: (03) 9726 9008
Western Australia	Phone: 1800 138 029

Chronic Illness Alliance Vic. (CIA) is an umbrella organisation that helps other organisations that support people with chronic illnesses. It provides regular newsletters to individual and group members:
818 Burke Road
Camberwell, Vic. 3124
Phone: (03) 9805 9126
Email: mail@chronicillness.org.au
Website: www.chronicillness.org.au

Books

The New People: Not Patients: A source book for living with inflammatory bowel disease
A useful book with plenty of pictures and illustrations. It covers the basics of IBD, including the emotional issues, and is published by the American Crohn's and Colitis Foundation.
Author: Dr Penny Steiner-Grossman
Publisher: Crohn's & Colitis Foundation of America, revised 1997

Managing Your Child's Crohn's disease or Ulcerative Colitis
The Australian Crohn's and Colitis Foundation recommends this book written by two esteemed paediatricians. It is described as 'a complete paediatric resource for parents and families' and it also includes chapters for teenagers.
Authors: Keith J. Benkov and Harland S. Winter
Publisher: Mastermedia Publishing Company, 1996

Ulcerative Colitis and Crohn's Disease: An overview of the diseases and their treatment
This is a free patient-information booklet available from your GP. The Falk Foundation produces it. It contains useful, up-to-date information without drug company advertising.

Authors: J. Scholmerich, H. Herfarth, G. Rogler and A. Furst
Publisher: Falk Foundation, 2005

Useful websites

The Crohn's and Colitis Foundation of America is a not-for-profit organisation that provides support and information for people with IBD. It has some very good pamphlets that can be downloaded from the website: www.ccfa.org.

The National Association for Colitis and Crohn's Disease (NACC) is a member-based patient organisation in the United Kingdom. The website has good information sheets to download on various topics: www.nacc.org.uk.

This UK website has some great pamphlets to download about living with IBD and FAQs. It also discusses children with IBD. You can find it at: www.ibdclub.org.uk.

Dietary information
To find an accredited dietitian in your state or territory, go to the Dietitians Association of Australia website. This site also has useful dietary tips and advice: www.daa.asn.au.

For tips on eating healthily and adding fibre to your diet, go to: www.betterhealth.vic.gov.au.

An online information service set up by Australian gastroenterologists and health professionals includes dietary information for IBD and other digestive disorders: www.gastro.net.au.

9
Diverticular disease

I have been getting a dragging sensation on my left side now for a few years, and noticed over the last few months that when I go to the toilet it looks like 'rabbit droppings'. Last month I had horrible abdominal pain, and felt hot and sweaty. My GP gave me antibiotics and that seemed to stop the pain after a day or so. He said I probably had diverticular disease and I had experienced an episode of diverticulitis. He has also organised for me to have a colonoscopy. He said it wasn't uncommon at my age, and told me to drink more water and eat more foods with fibre to lower the risk of another attack.

Margaret, 65, retired teacher

What is diverticular disease?

Diverticular disease, or **diverticulosis** as it is sometimes called, affects the large bowel and is characterised by little pockets forming in the bowel wall called **diverticula** (diverticulum is the singular). To picture it, think of the bowel as a bike tyre. Diverticula form when the tube bulges through the tyre because it is under too much pressure or the walls wear thin. A famous British surgeon, Sir Erasmus Wilson, is thought to have been the first to describe a diverticulum in about 1840. Sir Erasmus is best known for paying £10 000 to transport the famous monument, Cleopatra's Needle, from Egypt to London.

The reason why diverticula form is not really known, but it is more common in older people and people from Western societies. It has been found that diverticula are more likely to occur in people with low-fibre diets. It is believed that pressure builds up in the bowel and, if there is any weakness in the strength of the bowel wall, this pressure causes the mucosal layer of the large bowel to push through the muscle, creating the 'out pouch' or pocket. Constipation leads to straining and increased pressure in the bowel, which may make the formation of diverticula more likely. It usually occurs in the lower part of the large bowel in the sigmoid colon (see chapter one for more information on the bowel's anatomy), but can occur throughout the large bowel. Diverticula do not necessarily cause any problems and many people have diverticular disease without knowing it. Most people over the age of 60 have diverticular disease, but only a small proportion of people with the disease, about 10 per cent, go on to develop symptoms such as those of diverticulitis.

What is diverticulitis?

Diverticulitis is a local infection of one or more diverticula. The diverticula can become infected for many reasons and the inflammation from the infection can range from mild to severe. A common reason for the infection is that the undigested material passing through the large bowel gets stuck in one of the diverticula and causes a local inflammatory reaction. Bacterial overgrowth can also cause an infection of the diverticula, which fill up with pus. Diverticulitis can be severe and may require hospitalisation. In extreme cases where diverticulitis recurs and does not respond to treatment, surgery may be needed.

Figure 9.1 Diverticula in the large bowel

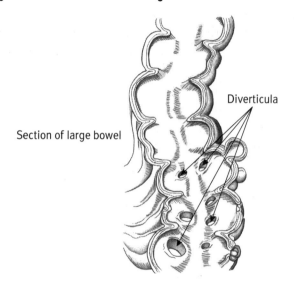

Diverticula

Section of large bowel

What are the symptoms of diverticular disease?

Symptoms vary depending on the cause and severity of the inflammation. Most people with diverticular disease have no symptoms. Others experience lower abdominal pain that is crampy, bloating, and an irregular bowel habit that can alternate between diarrhoea and constipation. Loss of appetite, nausea, flatulence (farting) and passing pellet-like stools can also be signs of diverticular disease. Rectal bleeding does not occur in uncomplicated diverticular disease.

Symptoms of diverticulitis include abdominal pain or cramps, often tenderness on the lower left side of the abdomen, fever and chills, nausea, occasionally vomiting, red blood in the stool or coming from the anus, diarrhoea and constipation.

Who gets diverticular disease?

Generally, it is older people from Western societies. The incidence of getting diverticula goes up with age. Half the population in Australia over the age of 80 will have diverticula. Societies with low-fibre diets have the highest incidence of diverticular disease. It is almost unheard of in Africa and parts of Asia where high-fibre diets are common. A British study in Oxford found that vegetarians, who have diets higher in fibre than non-vegetarians, had a one in ten chance of getting diverticular disease. This was much less than the one in three incidence rate of diverticular disease found in the non-vegetarian British population.

What causes diverticular disease?

It is not known what causes diverticular disease. As mentioned above, it is thought to be primarily caused by a low-fibre diet and a combination of factors that includes one or more of the following: chronic constipation and straining, genetic predisposition and ageing.

Fibre is the part of fruits, vegetables and grains that the body cannot digest. Fibre helps soften the stool and makes it easier to pass through the bowel. Fibre also prevents constipation. For more information on fibre, see chapter four on irritable bowel syndrome. Some experts also think that diverticular disease may be caused by a low-grade infection in the large bowel: This is still under evaluation.

Complications of diverticular disease

Complications can range from mild to severe. They can include diverticulitis, which may resolve with antibiotics, or may go on to cause an abscess. This may resolve also, but can lead to perforation and peritonitis. It may also lead to a fistula, which is a tunnel that tracks from the abscess and drains into the bladder or vagina or perianal skin. Sometimes scarring from the inflammation causes a narrowing of the bowel and this is known as a stricture: this may result in obstruction of the bowel.

Bleeding

Bleeding from diverticula is rare. Fresh red blood, rather than older brown blood, may appear in the toilet or in your stool. It may look like a lot of blood, but it usually stops by itself and does not require treatment other than a check-up. It is thought the bleeding is caused by small blood vessels in the diverticula that burst. If you have bleeding from the rectum, you should see your doctor so that it can be properly assessed. If a lot of blood has been lost, you may need a blood transfusion in hospital. Surgery is very uncommon for bleeding because it usually stops by itself. These days some specialists can treat ongoing bleeding from diverticular disease using a colonoscope. Very rarely, surgery is necessary to remove the affected bleeding bowel.

Abscess, perforation and peritonitis

An abscess forms when a diverticulum becomes infected (diverticulitis) and fills up with pus. A small abscess can often be treated successfully with oral antibiotics. If this doesn't work, it may need to be drained. The procedure used to drain it is called percutaneous catheter drainage and involves the doctor inserting a needle through the skin into the bowel. The needle is usually guided by an ultrasound or CT scan. This is a very successful and easily performed procedure. Rarely, surgery is needed to flush the abscess clean. If the infection is severe and has destroyed some of the bowel, the damaged area will need to be removed.

Sometimes the infected diverticula may burst causing a perforation. Through the perforation, pus can leak out of the colon into the abdominal area known as the peritoneum. Infection that spreads to this area is called peritonitis and can make you very sick. It needs surgery straightaway to flush out the abdominal cavity and remove the damaged part of the colon. Without surgery, peritonitis can be fatal.

Fistula

A fistula is an unintended tunnel that links one organ to another. Usually a diverticular fistula forms when a person with diverticulitis has an abscess and it erodes into an adjacent organ. Fistulas can form in many places, the most common are between the bowel and the vagina, bladder and the skin. Surgery is often needed to remove the fistula and the damaged part of the bowel where the fistula formed. To prevent further infection, the patient will need antibiotics via a drip and, depending on the location of the fistula, they might need a catheter to drain the bladder.

Intestinal obstruction

When the body fights an infection like diverticulitis, the healing process involves the formation of scar tissue. The scar tissue is usually less flexible than normal tissue in the area and can restrict the large intestine. In severe cases, scar tissue can cause a partial or total blockage of the large bowel. If this happens, the bowel is unable to work properly and undigested material cannot pass through. Surgery is needed to unblock the bowel. If the bowel is totally obstructed, the surgery must be done immediately.

How is diverticular disease diagnosed?

Diverticular disease can be difficult to diagnose because its symptoms mimic other GIT problems. Your doctor will want to take a personal history and feel your abdomen. They will ask about your symptoms and your bowel habits. They may order a blood test to see if you have general signs of infection, which could suggest diverticulitis. To confirm diagnosis, your doctor needs to be able to see the diverticula by ordering one of the tests below. For more detailed information on the tests, see chapter two.

Rectal examination

This involves lying on your side on a bed or trolley. Your doctor will insert a gloved, lubricated finger into your rectum. They are looking for any abnormal feeling of tenderness, a blockage, or blood. The procedure is quick and should take no more than a minute. It may be uncomfortable but is usually not painful.

Endoscopy (colonoscopy)

An endoscope is a narrow tube used to look inside the bowel. Most people these days have a colonoscopy or flexible sigmoid-oscopy. This involves inserting into the anus a soft, flexible tube with a TV camera and light at its end to get a view inside the bowel. A colonoscopy shouldn't be painful but you might feel pressure and slight cramping in your lower abdomen. In Australia, the procedure is done under light sedation, and there is usually no memory of the procedure after it is over.

A rigid sigmoidoscope

This is a shorter instrument that does not reach as far as the flexible sigmoidoscope. It goes only about 25 cm into the rectum via the anus. Its use is more limited and it is best for investigating the rectum. It is rarely ordered because colonoscopy often gives a better view, and is more comfortable.

CT scan

A CT (computed tomography) or CAT scan is an advanced type of X-ray that provides an inside view of the body. A special type of CT scan now available can give pictures similar to a colonoscopy (often called a CT colonoscopy or virtual colonoscopy). It has its limitations (you can't do biopsies) but it is good for detecting things like cancer and diverticulum.

Barium enema and X-ray

This test is used to get a picture of the inside of the colon. It is not so commonly done in Australia anymore since the advent of CT scanning, and the more common test is a colonoscopy. However, the barium enema is useful for seeing inflammation of the bowel, cancer and diverticular disease. It requires a bowel preparation, which involves drinking a clear fluid the night before.

Ultrasound

Also called sonography, an ultrasound is a method of getting images using high-frequency sound waves. The sound waves bounce off the organs and are recorded. Using a computer, the recordings are transferred into images. It is a good test for assessing organs that contain fluid. For this reason, if diverticulitis is suspected, the ultrasound may be able to pick up pus-filled diverticula.

If it is not diverticular disease, then what?

The two most important diagnoses to rule out when testing for diverticular disease are irritable bowel syndrome and bowel cancer. Not only do these conditions have similar symptoms, but bowel cancer also occurs in the elderly and can go undiagnosed for a long time because of the slow nature of the disease.

Table 9.1 Conditions that might be considered before diagnosing diverticulitis

Condition	*Symptoms	*Tests
Irritable bowel syndrome		
Abnormal sensitivity and coordination of muscle contraction in the bowel (see chapter four)	Cramping abdominal pain Nausea Bloating Diarrhoea and constipation	Gastroscopy Colonoscopy Blood tests
Cancer of the large bowel		
Abnormal cell growth in the large intestine	Abdominal pain Bleeding Weight loss	Blood test Colonoscopy
Inflammatory bowel disease		
Describes ulcerative colitis and Crohn's disease (see chapter eight)	Diarrhoea Abdominal pain Bleeding	Colonoscopy Blood tests
Urinary tract infections	Painful urination Abdominal pain Fever	Blood tests Urine analysis Abdominal X-rays

**Table 9.1 Conditions that might be considered before
diagnosing diverticulitis** *continued*

Condition	*Symptoms	*Tests
Gastroenteritis		
Stomach or bowel infection	Diarrhoea	Blood test
	Abdominal pain	Colonoscopy
	Vomiting	
Gynaecological conditions		
Ovarian cyst, endometriosis	Abdominal pain	Vaginal
	Abnormal bleeding	examination
	Discharge from the	Vaginal
	vagina	ultrasound
Appendicitis		
Inflamed or ruptured appendix	Abdominal pain	Surgery
	Fever	CT scan

*Note: Not all symptoms may be present; and not all tests may need to be ordered.

Treating diverticular disease

Many people with uncomplicated diverticular disease do not know they have it. Sometimes it is diagnosed when an unrelated problem is being investigated. For these people, a high-fibre diet is recommended to try and stop more diverticula forming. It is also important to drink lots of water to stop the stool drying out too much, which is a cause of constipation and can lead to straining—one of the theories of the cause of diverticula formation. The severity of the disease and its symptoms will determine the most appropriate treatment. All people with diverticular disease can benefit from the dietary changes recommended below. For mild diverticulitis being treated at home, a clear liquid or soft diet is recommended to give the bowel a rest. Pain relief and antibiotics will also be needed (see page 233). Severe diverticulitis will need to be managed in hospital.

Dietary changes—fibre

Increase the amount of fibre in your diet. You should be getting between 25 and 30 grams of fibre each day. To give you a better idea, this is equivalent to two pieces of fruit *and* five serves of vegetables (half a cup if cooked, one cup if raw) and four serves of either bread, cereal, grain or pasta made from whole grains (a serve is one cup; a serve of bread is two thin slices). Table 9.2 below gives you an idea of how much fibre is in some common foods.

Some high-fibre recipes have been included at the end of this book to help you with ideas about increasing the amount of fibre in your diet.

If you feel that you cannot get enough fibre through diet alone, you can use fibre supplements. They can be bought from a pharmacy or even your local health food store or supermarket. Examples include: Metamucil, Normafibe and Fybogel. These work by softening the stool and providing bulk. To work best, they need to be taken with plenty of water.

Drinking plenty of water is good advice anyway. Aim for at least 2 litres a day (seven to eight glasses). Other fluids, such as fruit juice, can also be counted; but remember that tea, coffee, cola soft drinks and alcohol are diuretics. This means that they stimulate the kidneys to pass more water and these fluids can actually make you more dehydrated. Avoid them if you can.

It was once thought to be a good idea to avoid tiny, hard food pieces like seeds, nuts and pips. The theory was that if these got stuck in the diverticula they could cause diverticulitis. However, no scientific studies have been able to support this theory. The most common cause of the development of diverticulitis is impacted faecal matter, not food. Therefore, dietary advice should focus on preventing constipation by eating high-fibre foods.

Table 9.2 What to eat—high-fibre foods

Fruits

Apple, raw, with skin	1 medium = 3.3 g
Peach, raw	1 medium = 1.5 g
Pear, raw	1 medium = 5.1 g

Vegetables

Asparagus, fresh, cooked	4 spears = 1.2 g
Broccoli, fresh, cooked	½ cup = 2.6 g
Brussels sprouts, fresh, cooked	½ cup = 2 g
Cabbage, fresh, cooked	½ cup = 1.5 g
Carrot, fresh, cooked	½ cup = 2.3 g
Cauliflower, fresh, cooked	½ cup = 1.7 g
Lettuce	1 cup = 1.2 g
Spinach, fresh, cooked	½ cup = 2.2 g
Summer squash, cooked	1 cup = 2.5 g
Tomato, raw	1 = 1 g
Winter squash, cooked	1 cup = 5.7 g

Starchy Vegetables

Baked beans, canned, plain	½ cup = 6.3 g
Kidney beans, fresh, cooked	½ cup = 5.7 g
Lima beans, fresh, cooked	½ cup = 6.6 g
Potato, fresh, cooked	1 = 2.3 g

Grain

Bread, whole-wheat	1 slice = 1.9 g
Brown rice, cooked	1 cup = 3.5 g
Cereal, bran flake	¾ cup = 5.3 g
Oatmeal, plain, cooked	¾ cup = 3 g
White rice, cooked	1 cup = 0.6 g

Drugs

Drugs do not change the long-term outlook of diverticular disease, however, they can be useful to treat complications and give short-term relief. These drugs are listed below.

Antibiotics

These need to be prescribed by your doctor. Some antibiotics can cause diarrhoea and make you feel nauseated. Some antibiotics need to be taken with food to minimise these side effects. Always finish the course of tablets (unless your doctor says otherwise). Even if you are feeling better, you will need to finish the course to make sure the infection has been properly treated.

Mild diverticulitis

A common antibiotic prescription for mild diverticulitis would be: amoxycillin 875 mg + clavulanate 125 mg taken orally, twice a day, for five to ten days. Other antibiotics can be used, such as metronidazole and cephalexin.

Severe diverticulitis

This needs to be managed and treated in hospital. People with severe diverticulitis usually improve within 48 to 72 hours. Initially they will be ordered not to have any food or fluids orally and will need bed rest. Fluids and antibiotics will be given intravenously via a drip, usually in the arm. Pain relief will also be necessary.

Analgesia (pain relief)

Severe diverticulitis can be very painful. In hospital, your doctor might prescribe an antispasmodic drug.

For mild diverticulitis being treated at home, you should take paracetamol every four hours. This will also help control a rising temperature.

Antispasmodic medications

These work by relaxing the muscle in the bowel wall, which can go into spasm because of the inflamed bowel. Occasionally these medications can cause a dry mouth. Examples include: Buscopan or Atrobel.

Surgery

Surgery is not needed in uncomplicated diverticular disease or uncomplicated diverticulitis. Surgery is *uncommon* and a last resort. The situations where surgery might be necessary include:

- **Severe diverticulitis**—If diverticulitis recurs several times in twelve months, elective surgery might be needed to prevent complications.
- **Diverticulitis with perforation**—This can be life threatening and will need emergency surgery to repair the leak.
- **Bleeding**—Bleeding from diverticular disease almost always stops by itself. Very rarely, surgery is used for life-threatening bleeding, and occasionally bleeding diverticula can also now be treated through a colonoscope.
- **Abscess**—If an abscess is unable to be properly drained by putting a catheter through the skin into the affected area, it may need immediate surgery to prevent peritonitis.
- **Fistula**—A fistula needs to be removed surgically, but it is rarely urgent.
- **Obstruction**—Where the bowel has become physically blocked because of scar tissue from recurrent diverticulitis, surgery will need to be done immediately.

The type of surgery performed will depend on a number of factors, including: the exact cause, the extent of bowel involved, how sick the patient is, and whether they had time to have a proper bowel preparation or not. When the surgery is elective, the bowel preparation involves drinking a clear fluid the day before the operation to get the bowel as clean and as empty as possible of faecal matter.

Elective surgery (with bowel preparation)

- **Resection and anastomosis**—This is an open operation that involves making a small lengthways cut across the abdomen, through the skin and through the muscle layers to reach the bowel. Then the affected part of the bowel is removed and the two healthy ends are rejoined to make the bowel one continuous pipe again. It is the most common bowel operation. For people with recurrent uncomplicated diverticulitis, this operation is the standard procedure performed. It is also used when patients have a fistula or an abscess.
- **Laparoscopic colectomy**—This is keyhole surgery. It involves making about three tiny cuts in the abdomen to remove the affected part of bowel. It is technically difficult to do and requires a skilled surgeon. It was first done in 1991 and surgeons are getting better at performing it. With an experienced surgeon, it is a safe operation and has the benefit of a much quicker recovery time.

Emergency surgery

- **Resection with sigmoid colostomy and closure of the rectal stump (Hartmann's procedure)**—A Hartmann's procedure is the most common surgery for emergency treatment of perforated diverticulitis. It involves two operations. The first is done immediately and involves cutting out the perforated area of the bowel. The bowel is then fashioned into a colostomy. This means that the bowel is attached to the abdominal wall and a new opening, called a **stoma**, is made in the skin. The stoma has a disposable bag attached to it, which catches the faecal matter. It is a temporary situation. Bags are changed after every bowel action. The patient will need this temporary bag for three to six months. Then, once the bowel has had a good chance to heal and recover, the stoma is removed and the bowel is reattached internally to the rectum. The procedure was named after the French surgeon who devised it, Henri Hartmann. For more information on stomas and their management see chapter eleven.

- **Transverse colostomy and drainage**—This procedure is rarely performed these days and is usually only done when peritonitis is so severe that it is unsafe to cut out the perforated segment of bowel. It involves opening the bowel, through the skin, with a stoma mid way along the large bowel. This takes pressure off the bowel lower down in an emergency situation when it is too dangerous to perform a larger operation.

Prognosis

Most people who suffer an episode of diverticulitis never have a repeat episode, and often attacks are only mild and can be treated with oral antibiotics. Surgery is uncommon and is reserved for people with severe, recurrent diverticulitis or the complications of diverticular disease that have been outlined above.

Follow-up care for diverticulitis

After an episode of diverticulitis, you should have a follow-up colonoscopy or barium enema to see the extent of diverticular disease, and to exclude any other underlying problems such as a cancer. The good news is that less than a third of people who suffer uncomplicated diverticulitis will have a recurrent attack.

If a second and third attack occurs within a year, your doctor may discuss elective surgery. The surgery aims to remove some of the bowel where the diverticula are getting infected to prevent a major attack later that might need emergency surgery when the patient is very unwell. This is done about eight weeks after a severe episode.

Some common questions about diverticular disease

I am 61 and have been told that I have mild diverticular disease. Have I left it too late to start a high-fibre diet?

Studies of Vietnam soldiers suggest that many people already have diverticular disease in their 30s. There is some evidence to suggest a high-fibre diet will help prevent attacks of diverticulitis, so it is probably never too late to start. It may also have other health benefits, such as lowering cholesterol.

My twin brother and I have both been told that we have diverticular disease? Did we inherit this problem?

The jury is still out on whether diverticular disease is caused by diet, genetic factors, or perhaps even a low-grade infection. There probably is at least some inherited component responsible.

After having two episodes of severe diverticulitis, I am scared I might get bowel cancer. Is there an increased risk of cancer?

Probably not. One study performed suggested there may be a very slight increase in risk of cancer in people with diverticular disease, but the medical community does not generally accept this.

I get horrible cramps from diverticular disease. I have used an antispasmodic drug to try and stop the pain, but sometimes it feels like it makes the problem worse. Is this possible?

Experiencing spasm is not unusual in diverticular disease, and is probably caused by scarring that occurs after a bout of diverticulitis.

This leads to narrowing in the bowel which can then be stretched, causing the muscle to spasm.

My sister was admitted to hospital with diverticulitis. She was diagnosed with diverticulosis about four years ago. Is this the same thing?

No. Diverticulosis refers to having diverticula in your bowel. If these become infected, this is described as diverticulitis. Most people with diverticulosis never go on to get diverticulitis.

Further information

Medical contacts

Gastroenterological Society of Australia (GESA)
145 Macquarie Street
Sydney NSW 2000
Phone: (02) 9256 5454
Fax: (02) 9241 4586
Email: gesa@gesa.org.au
Website: www.gesa.org.au

British Society of Gastroenterology
3 St Andrews Place
Regents Park
London NW1 4LB
Phone: +44 (0) 20 7935 3150
Fax: +44 (0) 20 7487 3734
Email: bsg@mailbox.ulcc.ac.uk
Website: www.bsg.org.uk

American College of Gastroenterology official patient information website: www.acg.gi.org/patients/patientinfo/gerd.asp.

American Gastroenterological Association (AGA)
National Office
4930 Del Ray Avenue
Bethesda, MD 20814
Phone: +1 (301) 654 2055
Fax: +1 (301) 654 5920
Email: members@gastro.org
Website: www.gastro.org

Books

Good Gut Cook Book
Australian dietitian Rosemary Stanton and The Gut Foundation have teamed up to create a book of recipes for people with GIT problems including diverticular disease.
　　Authors: Rosemary Stanton and The Gut Foundation
　　Publisher: HarperHealth, 1998

Useful websites

A handy factsheet on diverticulitis can be found on the GESA Website: www.gesa.org.au/leaflets/diverticulitis.cfm.

CORE, formerly Digestive Disorders Foundation is the official UK health website on GIT problems that includes information on diverticulosis: www.corecharity.org.uk.

The National Digestive Diseases Information Clearinghouse (NDDIC) is a US government health information service. Its website has useful information for sufferers of digestive diseases: http://digestive.niddk.nih.gov/ddiseases/pubs/diverticulosis.

The Mayo Clinic is one of America's top medical research centres. You can download patient information on diverticular disease at its website: www.mayoclinic.com/health/diverticulitis/ DS00070.

Dietary information

The Gut Foundation is an Australian organisation that provides professional and public education, and promotes research into digestive disorders to improve gastrointestinal health: www.gut. nsw.edu.au.

You can also find an accredited dietitian in your state or territory by contacting the Dietitians Association of Australia (DAA). Its website also has useful dietary tips and advice: www. daa.asn.au.

This useful Victorian government health website has information on eating healthily for people suffering different diseases, including diverticular disease: www.betterhealth.vic.gov.au.

10
More about treatments

The role of alternative therapies

This book is primarily focused on conventional, evidence-based medicine. This refers to the scientific way that doctors and scientists find answers to problems. At the research level, they do this by gathering and studying information and subjecting it to statistical analysis in order to disprove or support a theory. The process of determining a diagnosis is similar; it starts with collecting information and making an informed judgement based on their findings. Doctors must comply with scientific principles in order to have their findings published, and earn the respect of peers and the wider medical community. This does not mean that the process is infallible. Everyone is capable of making mistakes and test results can be wrongly interpreted. There are also famous cases where doctors have fraudulently altered the results to get a favourable outcome.

One example was that of Dr William McBride, the Australian doctor made famous for his important discovery of the link between birth defects and the morning sickness drug thalidomide.

Unfortunately, years later his scientific standards slipped and he was deregistered from working as a medical researcher for falsifying results to speed up his research into birth defects. He was allowed to continue working as a doctor.

Alternative or complementary medicines do not fit the same medical model as conventional medicine. Their approach relies on a combination of intuition and test methods that may not be recognised by the scientific community. These techniques may include assessing a person's tongue, feet or eyes to make judgements about the overall health of the body and mind. One of the comforting things that alternative therapists do is look at the person as a whole and not just as a diseased bowel, which is the impression some medical doctors can give in their apparent haste. This recognition restores a patient's dignity and can help someone who has been sick regain a sense of control over their life and their illness.

Unfortunately, as in all walks of life, there are occasionally profiteers in alternative therapies who exploit patients' interest and offer people false hope where none exists. Also, words like 'natural' and 'cure' are sometimes abused. Just because something occurs naturally does not mean it is safe. For example, the Chinese herb Jin Bu Huan, used as a sedative and pain reliever, can cause liver failure.

There is a role for alternative therapies in the treatment of disease. If you are interested in this path, don't be discouraged by the friction you may encounter between some conventional doctors and alternative therapists because of their different approaches to illness, diagnosis and treatment. Some doctors can be defensive if you want to try an alternative therapy because they are concerned that you will jeopardise your health by foregoing a well-tested conventional treatment for the sake of an unproven therapy that could be harmful.

Some complementary medicine practitioners are trying to ease these tensions by embracing the tools of conventional medicine. They are doing evidence-based studies to get wider recognition for their therapies. Also, some therapists are making use of the diagnostic equipment of conventional doctors, such as the blood pressure machine, X-rays and so on to help with their work. Conversely, some doctors are studying alternative medicines to offer their patients more options in the treatment of their illnesses. Also, some of the principles of alternative medicines are very complementary to conventional medicine such as the emphasis on good nutrition, drinking lots of water, changing your lifestyle to reduce stress, and avoiding habits that harm you such as smoking and an excessive intake of alcohol. Many of my patients find yoga and massage particularly helpful in the treatment of the symptoms of irritable bowel syndrome. The bottom line is, whether the treatment you consider is conventional or alternative, use your judgement and be aware of quackery. Almost never is there a quick fix for a chronic illness. Research the treatments you are interested in and don't be taken in by labels that promise miracles.

What are alternative therapies?

Alternative therapies, also called natural therapies or complementary medicine, have been around since ancient times. This umbrella term covers hundreds of different treatments including massage, Chinese herbal medicine, homeopathy, reiki (healing through touch), acupuncture and yoga. Some therapies were copied from the practices of shamans, witch-doctors, Eastern healing traditions, and the healing practices of American Indians and other ancient civilisations of Egypt, Greece and Rome.

Alternative therapies have become popular in the Western world. Some therapies are modern developments, such as homeopathy which was founded at the beginning of the nineteenth century. Broadly speaking, alternative therapies are divided into three broad categories (some may overlap):

- **Physical**—These work on the body, such as chiropractic and massage.
- **Psychological**—These focus on the mind to heal the body, such as meditation, counselling and hypnotherapy.
- **Energy**—These are Eastern traditions that believe the body has energy flows, which are interrupted when we get unwell. Therapies that focus on energy include acupuncture and shiatsu.

Alternative therapists do not always agree with one another. For example, some would not recommend colonic irrigation, which involves inserting a tube into the rectum to flush the bowel with warm water to remove faecal matter—because of the potential danger of perforating the bowel and upsetting the balance of normal bowel bacteria. Most medical doctors also have this viewpoint. However, if you needed to decipher some common principles, most therapies subscribe to the idea that:

- The body has an amazing ability to heal itself.
- You need to take control of your situation and take on a positive role by changing lifestyle and habits.
- Health is a complex phenomenon that involves a balance between the body, mind and spirit.
- Our environment and social situation affect our health.
- An overriding healing force exists in the universe, which can be mustered to help restore health.
- Therapists need to treat the underlying cause, not just the symptoms.

With these principles in mind, your therapist will want to understand you as much as your symptoms. They may want to see you for up to an hour on your first visit to get a holistic understanding of your problem. You may be asked questions about all aspects of your health and life, including sleep patterns, lifestyle, social life, past health problems and diet.

It is not possible to discuss in detail in this book all the alternative therapy options, so an overview of the more common therapies used to treat gastrointestinal disorders has been outlined. This book does not endorse any particular therapy and recommends that if you are interested in alternative therapies, you should talk to your doctor about it first. Information on finding qualified alternative therapists is given later in this chapter.

Acupressure

According to ancient Chinese practice, the body is said to have energy fields and these run along twelve meridian lines that map the body. Acupressure is applying pressure to particular points along the meridian lines to regulate the flow of energy, called Chi. These are the same points used in acupuncture but, instead of using needles, acupressure relies on fingertip or fingernail pressure. Occasionally round-ended wooden sticks are used. Once learned, it is a good self-help technique. To be effective, acupressure needs to be done daily for a few minutes, usually in a circular motion. Shiatsu is the Japanese variant of acupressure. For GIT problems, acupressure is sometimes recommended to treat constipation and diarrhoea by relieving stress. It is also used to relieve the pain of stomach ache, indigestion and ulcers, and to treat faecal incontinence. See a qualified acupressurist for more information.

Acupuncture

This therapy has great appeal to some Western medical practitioners who are learning the therapy as an adjunct to conventional treatments. It was first practised in China more than 5000 years ago. It was positively reviewed in a leading British medical journal in 1827 and has been used in the UK and across Europe since. It is recognised by the World Health Organisation and is now practised in most parts of the developed world. Like acupressure, acupuncture involves working with the 350 pressure points along the meridian lines. Each line correlates with an organ or system. Fine sterile needles are inserted into the selected points to help the flow of energy (Chi). The needles are so fine that they do not usually cause pain and the aim is to restore balance to the opposing forces of energy, yin and yang. It is reported that a feeling of relaxation quickly follows. The needles are left in place for a short time, and may be gently moved, rotated or flicked to help energy flows. For GIT complaints, acupuncture can be used to treat constipation and diarrhoea caused by stress, and IBS and IBD symptoms, and to relieve constipation in diverticulitis. Visit a qualified acupuncturist for more information.

Aromatherapy

This is the use of plant oils (essential oils) and their perfumes to influence the body to improve health. Some oils are used to relax the body, others are used to stimulate the body and make the mind more alert. Some are said to have antibacterial, anti-inflammatory and pain-relieving effects. If diluted in a base oil, such as almond oil, they can be applied directly to the skin, massaged into the body, and inhaled either via a vaporiser or by breathing in the steam from a bowl of hot water containing the oil. Some people also like to put essential oils in the bath. Ten commonly used essential oils are: chamomile (calming), eucalyptus (pain relieving), geranium (healing), lavender (pain relieving), rose (antiseptic), rosemary (mild stimulant), sandalwood (antiseptic), marjoram (pain relieving), jasmine (antidepressant), and neroli (sedative). In treating the GIT, peppermint oil can be taken to treat indigestion. A bath containing peppermint oil or chamomile oil is used to treat the pain of haemorrhoids. Inhaled peppermint oil is also used to treat the pain of IBS. Lavender oil is the choice for symptoms of IBD. Marjoram oil in cooking is used to limit flatulence. Aromatherapy is not recommended during pregnancy. See a qualified aromatherapist for more information.

Herbal medicine

As the name suggests, this therapy involves the use of herbs to treat ailments and improve health. It is an ancient form of treatment used by most civilisations at some time, probably starting with the Egyptians. They learned which herbs and plants had a healing effect through trial and error. Some drugs today contain herbal extracts or are derived from plants, such as the powerful heart drug, digoxin, which comes from the leaves of *Digitalis purpurea*, better known as the flower, foxglove. Like some other herbs, it can be deadly and is poisonous in its raw form. Herbs should never be underestimated for their potentially toxic effects on the body and should never be taken without expert advice. Herbs can affect the workings of most parts of the body including the digestive system. Herbs as treatments can come in many forms including ointments, lozenges, creams, tablets, skin compresses and tinctures. Herbalists use herbal treatments in the digestive system to treat nausea, gastroenteritis, hangovers, coeliac disease, indigestion, heartburn, stomach ache, constipation, diarrhoea and haemorrhoids. Chamomile, peppermint, fennel and other herbs are used to relieve the symptoms of IBS.

Homeopathy

The founder of homeopathy in the nineteenth century was a German doctor and chemist, Samuel Hahnemann. A monument dedicated to his life and work stands in Washington DC. By chance Hahnemann noted that the compound quinine used to treat malaria actually produced the symptoms of malaria in healthy people. Using this principle of *like cures like* he experimented with popular medicines to find out their toxic effects on healthy individuals, then diluted and prepared minute doses for sick people who presented with similar symptoms. In 1810, he wrote a book about his findings, *Organon of the Healing Art*, and his theories and methods are still used today. Homeopathy is used to treat some digestive disorders including gastroenteritis, nausea, stomach ache, indigestion, hangover, diarrhoea, constipation, faecal incontinence, haemorrhoids, inflammation of the bowel, and ulcers. See a qualified homeopath for more information.

Reflexology

Reflexology is based on the belief that our health is reflected in the soles of our feet. It identifies reflex points on the feet (and sometimes hands and ears) that are said to correspond with the organs in one of ten mapped zones of the body. For example, the big toe correlates with the head, the left foot corresponds with the left side of the body, and so on. By massaging these points, it is thought to promote healing of organs belonging to the corresponding zone and generate overall wellness. Two Americans, Eunice Ingham and Dr William Fitzgerald, adapted the modern use of reflexology from ancient techniques practised by American Indians, Egyptians and Grecians. Reflexology is used in the GIT to help relieve diarrhoea and constipation.

Relaxation techniques

There are many different types of relaxation techniques but their purpose is the same: to calm the mind and body to promote good health. The idea is that if the body and mind are in a relaxed state, they can get on with healing themselves. There are other benefits too—greater mental alertness, a feeling of contentment, easing of pain, and stress reduction. Relaxation is an enjoyable state and can be practised in a group class. Some of the methods to achieve relaxation include yoga, massage, meditation and biofeedback. Yoga is terrific for strengthening core body muscles. Biofeedback uses technology to give feedback about the body's responses, such as heart rate and respiratory rate, so that a conscious effort can be made to slow down your breathing and relax. Relaxation is thought to be good for many digestive problems, particularly IBS and IBD. To learn various relaxation techniques, see a qualified instructor.

How to find a skilled therapist

If you want to try an alternative therapy, find someone who is properly qualified. If you are acting on a friend's recommendation or have found a phone number in the telephone book, don't be afraid to ask the therapist about their formal qualifications and whether they are a member of a governing association. If they are professionals, they won't mind you asking. A reliable way to find a skilled practitioner is to ring the nearest major training college; there are more than 170 across Australia. Most of these institutions offer services to the public and are happy to recommend therapists in the different disciplines. You can also get a directory of therapists from the relevant association.

Changing your lifestyle

Medical science has now shown that stress is not a primary cause of stomach ulcers as once thought, however, lifestyle choices and stress can have a negative impact on a number of chronic GIT disorders. The influence of stress on the digestive system is discussed below.

Stress and the GIT

Research and anecdotal evidence have found that there is a link between stress, particularly chronic stress, and some GIT disorders such as IBS. Studies in the 1960s first found that major stressful life events, such as divorce, separation, moving house and even positive events like marriage and holidays, often occurred just before the onset of bowel symptoms. These findings have been repeated in newer studies, some finding that chronic stress influenced the onset and duration of bowel symptoms in four out of five women and one in three men. Chronic stress included events such as relationship difficulties, serious illness, lawsuits, business failure, housing problems, being sacked or demoted at work, and caring for a sick relative. Other studies have found that when these stressors are resolved or stress-management skills are employed, there has been an improvement in bowel symptoms.

Stress—what is it?

Stress is a hard concept to pin down. It can physically and emotionally affect us. Physically, a stressful event can stimulate the nervous and hormonal systems to prepare the primordial 'fight or flight' response. Significant stress can create hyperactivity in the intestines, which can cause diarrhoea or, in extreme cases, loss of control of our bowels. Emotionally, stress can leave us feeling tired, negative, depressed and anxious. But stress is not always negative. The tension we feel before giving a public performance, or sitting an exam, can be used positively and can improve our performance by sharpening our reflexes and mind. Stress can cause the release of adrenaline and other chemicals that can leave us feeling excited and euphoric. But how we respond to a potentially stressful event can be difficult to predict. The same event can have different impacts on different people. It depends on our ability to cope with a situation, and that may depend on our genetics, personality, previous experiences, learned coping skills and so on. One of the modern researchers on stress, the late American psychologist Professor Richard Lazarus, argued that stress and coping were closely connected. He found that people experience stress if they think they do not have the resources to manage difficult events. Conversely they do not suffer stress if they believe that they have such resources. If he is right, it means that, to some degree, we may be able to reduce the amount of stress *we feel* in our lives by improving our coping mechanisms. This is good news because stress will always exist in some form, whether it be a parking ticket, running late for work, or an illness. Some ways in which we can do that are detailed below. But first, it is important to identify the stress in your life.

Identifying stress

If you are stressed, you may be experiencing any number of these things:

- Mood swings
- Anxiety
- Skin problems
- Tiredness
- Muscle tension
- Poor concentration
- Changes in sleep patterns
- Changes in eating patterns
- Low self-esteem
- Poor memory.

To reduce stress, you need to be able to recognise it. There are a number of ways you can do this. Keep a diary. Whenever you feel stressed, write it down. You need to be really honest with yourself and rank the stress you feel from zero to ten. Ten is the rating you would give to the worst stress imaginable, and zero is complete relaxation. If you are experiencing physical symptoms, make a note of these too, even if at the time you think that they are unrelated. When you are feeling stressed, write down possible reasons why and what actions you took. Make a note of whether these actions improved the situation or made it worse. After a few weeks, reflect on what you have written. You might see a pattern emerging that shows you the types of things that stress you and whether your management techniques are successful or not. Use this information to understand how your body responds to stress and when it occurs. This will help you prepare to manage stress.

There are questionnaires that you can do about stress and life events that will give you a point score at the end. The higher the score, the more stress you have. Although these life-event tests are freely available on the Internet, they are probably best done with the supervision of a psychologist who can ensure they are interpreted correctly for you.

Another way to identify stress is to draw up some columns to list what you think are your strengths, weaknesses, opportunities and threats. Organisations regularly do this type of analysis to help a business grow. In the strengths column, include things like your support network, financial resources, skills and past experiences. In the weaknesses column, be honest and think of what you are not so good at: write down any limitations of resources that you think impact on your ability to better manage your life. For example, is education, money or housing options a significant limiting factor on your choices in life to date? Just recognising a difficulty can be the first step to overcoming it. Be fair to yourself. In the opportunities column, list positive things that the future may hold for you and the reasons why. In the threats column, think about the consequences of what can happen if you don't address your weaknesses. Now you have developed a blueprint for change. Work at strengthening your weaknesses and build on your strengths to achieve your goals and work towards making the opportunities a reality.

Stress management

Changing the way we think about stress is one way to improve our health and peace of mind. Psychologists specialising in cognitive behaviour therapy can be particularly helpful in helping you to work on this long-term goal.

Hypnotherapy can also play a role in stress management and bowel symptoms. A British study of patients with IBS who underwent a course of hypnotherapy found that 65 per cent experienced an improvement in their bowel function after three months. The results of this study have been repeated in subsequent trials.

In the meantime, there are lifestyle changes you can do immediately to improve your health and help combat stress.

Quit smoking

If you are a smoker, try and give it up. It will make you feel fitter and you may be better able to cope with stress. Ring the Quitline or visit the website for a free brochure pack on different methods for quitting: www.quit.org.au.

Limit tea, coffee and alcohol intake

Caffeine stimulates the body and can speed up the GIT, sometimes causing loose bowel actions. Alcohol is a depressant. More than two glasses a day can adversely affect your mood, internal bodily functions and physical performance.

Exercise

Physical exercise increases our heart rate, blood flow to our brains and vital organs, and our metabolism. It can help us lose weight and it allows fat tissue to be converted to muscle tissue. Exercise stimulates the release of feel-good hormones called endorphins, so that we feel a sense of wellbeing afterwards. Try to do some type of exercise for about 20 minutes at a time, three or four times a week. Try to be realistic and incorporate it into your everyday life so that it isn't just a fad. Exercise needs to be done regularly to be of benefit. You can do this by walking or riding a bike to work. If it is too far, walk to the second-closest train or bus stop. Take the dog for a walk in the evening. Join a sporting club, enrol in a gym and follow a program, or get out and do some work in the garden. Decide what is going to suit your needs best and aim to stick with it for a few months; you may be surprised at how good you feel by the end of that trial period.

Sleep

Sleep is a critical time for our body to repair itself and refresh our mind. It is obvious when children don't get enough sleep. Their behaviour deteriorates; they can become moody, emotional and irrational. Adults are no different, but the signs are much more subtle. As sleep-deprived adults, we are able to mask the extremes; instead of tears, we may be a bit short-tempered with other people or we may feel irritable and tense. When we are tired, we are more vulnerable to feeling stressed. Nothing cures tiredness like sleep. Most adults need between seven and eight hours a day. Some people can cope well with as little as five, while others need ten. Pregnant women need more in the first three months. As we get older, we tend to need less. But, when we miss out on sleep, we develop a sleep-debt. Studies have found that people who do shift work can get particularly sleep deprived. This can impair their mental function in much the same way as alcohol does. We can avoid this by repaying the debt and catching up on sleep during the day, having a siesta, or going to bed early at night. A good night's sleep can help us see problems more positively in the morning.

A well-balanced diet

Generally speaking, lots of fresh fruit and vegetables high in fibre and drinking 2 litres of water a day is a good basis for a healthy diet (see chapter one). Also, just as regular sleep is important to our body functions, so are regular meals. Don't skip meals and try to avoid relying on takeaway food that is high in saturated fat.

Relaxation techniques

Feeling relaxed and content not only makes life enjoyable, but it also has positive effects on our health, including our bowels. Try and find some time each day to relax and unwind without the pressure of any commitments. You may want to find a therapy to help you relax. A simple, easy relaxation technique is breathing exercises. Just breathing in slowly, holding your breath for ten seconds and exhaling slowly can help you feel less tense. Some other options that you may want to consider include massage, meditation and floatation. The latter is when you float in a purpose-built floatation tank. Another relaxation technique— taught by psychotherapists—is visualisation; this is where you close your eyes and visualise a pleasant relaxed place, or a positive outcome to a situation that is causing you stress.

Emotional support

Surround yourself with people that care about you. This may include family, friends, colleagues or even pets. The old adage that 'a problem shared is a problem halved' is often true. Friends and family may help you see another perspective to a situation that you hadn't considered. The warmth of a good friend or relative is wonderful for our sense of wellbeing, as is being intimate with our partner. Sex is a great de-stressor. If you live away from family and friends, consider joining a social or interest group. A regular meeting with some like-minded people can be a good way to make new friends and to distract you from your own problems. If you are looking for someone to talk to about specific health problems, see if there is a support group nearby, or look at the resource section at the end of each chapter to find credible websites where you can read about others' coping techniques.

But, a word of caution, never give private details such as bank account numbers, phone numbers or addresses through an unsecured site on the Internet. You never know who might see them or how they might be used.

Further information

Useful contacts

To quit smoking, phone the **Quitline** for help, telephone 13 78 48 in Australia; or visit www.quit.org.au

Australian College of Natural Medicine
Website: www.acnm.edu.au

Queensland
362 Water St
Fortitude Valley Qld 4006
Phone: (07) 3257 1883
Fax: (07) 3257 1889

1 Nerang Street
Southport Qld 4215
Phone: (07) 5503 0977
Fax: (07) 5503 0988

Victoria
368 Elizabeth Street
Melbourne Vic. 3000
Phone: (03) 9662 9911
Fax: (03) 9662 9414

2A Cambridge Street
Box Hill Vic. 3128

Phone: (03) 9890 5599
Fax: (03) 9898 8260

Western Australia
170 Wellington Street
East Perth WA 6004
Phone: (08) 9225 2900
Fax: (08) 9225 2999

Books

Cambridge Handbook of Psychology, Health and Medicine
A thorough book with information on various alternative thera-
pies and the psychological aspects of coping with an illness.
 Editors: Andrew Baum, Stanton Newman, John Weinman,
 Robert West and Chris McManus
 Publisher: Cambridge University Press, 1997
 Available in major book stores.

Prescription for Dietary Wellness: Using foods to heal
A bestseller in the United States, this book looks at every aspect of
nutrition and provides scores of recipes. Note, however, that some
of the detox information is controversial by conventional medical
standards.
 Authors: James F. Balch and Phyllis A. Balch
 Publisher: Avery, 1998, 2nd edition
 Available at: www.amazon.com

The Healthy Living Book
Produced by Nutrition Australia, this great resource book helps
you to learn about eating healthily and how to be more physically
active. It is also very affordable.
 Author: Nutrition Australia
 Publisher: Nutrition Australia, 2005
 Available at: www.nutritionaustralia.org

Stress, Coping and Social Support in the Age of Anxiety
Dr Antony Kidman is a clinical psychologist and director of the Health Psychology Unit at the University of Technology, Sydney. In this book he provides some practical advice on coping with stress in your life.
  Author: Dr Antony Kidman, AM
  Publisher: Foundation for Life Sciences, 2005
  Available at: Foundation for Life Sciences
  Phone: (02) 9438 3828

Useful websites

Natural Therapy Pages: this commercial telephone and web directory helps you find therapists across Australia: www.naturaltherapy pages.com.au.

Austherapy: this is another useful commercial directory with a listing of schools and colleges: www.austherapy.com.au.

If you want some critical analysis of the therapies, go to the American Skeptics dictionary for a counter perspective: http:// skepdic.com.

The International Stress Management Association UK is a registered charity with a multi-disciplinary professional membership: www.isma.org.uk.

Nutrition Australia is a not-for-profit, non-government, community-based organisation that aims to educate the population about healthy eating and living: www.nutritionaustralia.org.

11
Living with a stoma

I have been struggling with ulcerative colitis for most of my teenage years. I have about twenty bowel actions a day and the pain is sometimes almost too much to bear. My disease is active nearly all the time and my doctor has suggested I have my large bowel removed and a J-pouch formed. He said I would need to have a temporary ileostomy for about six weeks to give my bowel time to heal. I am scared, but my doctor tells me I will be basically cured after the surgery. I have met the stoma therapist and she says at my age I can expect to live a long, healthy life. So, I am now starting to look forward to the idea of being free of ulcerative colitis.

Jane, 22, student

These days, very few Australians need to have a permanent stoma. Of the stomas that are fashioned, 70 per cent are temporary stomas that have been put in place usually to give the bowel time to heal after surgery. Colorectal surgery and the appliances available to manage a stoma have also improved enormously in the last few decades. This has meant that living with a stoma has been made easier. Rae Bourke, a clinical nurse consultant and stoma therapist at the Royal Melbourne Hospital, says that people living with a stoma can still enjoy good health, an active sex life, full-term pregnancy, working a difficult job or raising a family. In other words, life does not have to change too much. How you cope with a stoma is going to depend on your attitude and ability to accept it and get on with life.

In her clinical experience, Rae finds that how well someone copes with a stoma depends on their age, personal background, personality, the disease necessitating surgery, and the facilities and resources available to help people cope after surgery.

How you cope with a stoma is largely up to you. So find out as much as you can before the operation. Don't be afraid to ask your surgeon everything you want to know about the operation beforehand. Think carefully about where you want your stoma to be positioned on your body and tell your stoma therapist. Your choices may be limited, but it is worth expressing your opinion because you have to be able to live with your stoma. Also, think about the types of clothes you wear so that the stoma is not right on your belt line or too conspicuous above your jeans.

What is a stoma?

A stoma is a surgically created opening from anywhere in the large or small bowel, but more often in the large bowel which brings the bowel out to the skin. Its function is to allow waste products, faecal material, to leave the body. 'Stoma' means 'mouth' in Greek. A stoma, also called an ostomy, is made when either the small bowel or large bowel is unable to work properly. This can be for many reasons, such as cancer, bowel obstruction, a hereditary disease such as familiar polyposis, IBD, an abnormality since birth, and trauma. In a minority of cases, the stoma is permanent. In IBD, a temporary stoma may be fashioned to 'cure' ulcerative colitis (some patients may still have extra-intestinal symptoms so cure is used here in reference to bowel symptoms only). Stomas are less common in the treatment of Crohn's disease: this is because doctors try to avoid removing the bowel unless it is necessary as there is no cure for Crohn's disease and so the goal is to preserve whatever healthy bowel there is. Very occasionally, a temporary stoma may be made if a diseased part of the bowel needs to be removed: this is to protect the new internal surgical join (anastomosis) until it has had time to heal. No two stomas are alike because they vary depending on their location in the bowel, the surgeon's technique and the individual patient. But all stomas should be pink and moist (like the inside of your mouth), and they should not be painful. A stoma does not have a valve like the sphincter in the anal canal, so there is no control over when it will eliminate the body's waste from the bowel. For this reason, a pouch, sometimes called an appliance, is worn over the stoma to catch the bowel's output.

There are two main types of stomas: a colostomy and an ileostomy. The main type of stoma used in IBD is an ileostomy. Colostomy surgery is usually done to treat cancer of the bowel; it is rarely performed for IBD. Most people with colostomies are middle-aged or older, while temporary ileostomies can be found in all age groups. Temporary loop ileostomies are more common in Australia today than permanent colostomies as they are often fashioned to protect an anastomosis or join.

What is a colostomy?

A colostomy is a surgically created opening that is made in the large bowel. It can be made at almost any point along the bowel. A colostomy is usually placed on the abdomen on the lower left side. There are three types of colostomies: an end colostomy (usually permanent); a loop colostomy (usually temporary); and a transverse colostomy (this may sit up higher on the right side of the abdomen). Colostomies are rarely used to treat IBD. Occasionally, they may be needed temporarily if the bowel becomes obstructed and a section of bowel needs to be removed.

Figure 11.1 A colostomy

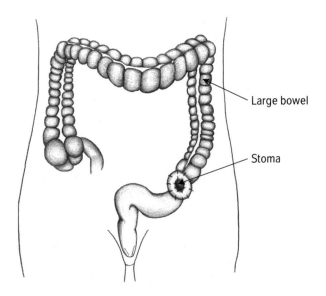

The waste matter from a colostomy is usually a formed stool, although occasionally some people may experience chronic diarrhoea or hard pellets. Constipation can also be a problem for some people with a colostomy if they fail to eat adequate amounts of fibre or take some medications.

What is an ileostomy?

An ileostomy is a surgically created opening that is made in the last section of the small intestine, called the terminal ileum. It is usually placed on the lower right side of the abdomen. There are three types of ileostomies: a loop ileostomy (usually temporary); an end ileostomy (usually permanent); and a Koch ileostomy (permanent, but not done in Australia these days). In most cases, about 90 per cent, ileostomies are temporary and are done to protect a surgical join (an anastomosis) in the bowel after surgery. In IBD, an ileostomy and total colectomy may be considered for *severe* ulcerative colitis. This involves removing the large bowel. As ulcerative colitis does not attack the small bowel, this procedure is effectively a cure of the disease and the ileostomy is permanent.

The waste matter from an ileostomy is usually of a toothpaste-like consistency. The normal volume is between 500 and 800 ml over 24 hours. Because of the enzymes it contains, the output can irritate the surrounding skin (peristomal skin) if it touches it. If your stoma appliance fits properly, this should not happen.

What is a J-pouch?

One of the reasons that permanent end ileostomies are fewer in number today than 25 years ago is because of advancements in surgical techniques. One development has been the ileo anal pouch anastomosis, often called a J-pouch or ileal reservoir. This surgical procedure removes the whole of the large intestine in people with severe ulcerative colitis or familial polyposis coli, which is sometimes called familial adenomatous polyposis. In this procedure, a pouch is fashioned from the small intestine and it acts as a reservoir in the absence of the large bowel.

This surgery is most encouraging because people are able to be rid of their disease, yet remain faecally continent without the need of a permanent ileostomy.

Surgery is usually done as a two-stage procedure, but it can be done as a one- or three-stage operation depending on the patient's condition. The majority of patients may require a temporary stoma for three to six months.

Following surgery, patients may experience up to fifteen bowel actions per day. Once the stoma has been reversed, this number slowly decreases to five to ten per day in the following weeks. Some patients may only experience three to five bowel actions a day but this usually takes some months to achieve.

Rae Bourke recommends the strict use of barrier creams around the anus for the first few months after every bowel action to protect the skin from excoriation (burning) following J-pouch formation. An excellent protective cream is wool fat or lanolin; both are readily available and affordable. Drugs can be taken to thicken the faecal output if persistent diarrhoea is a problem or if the output fails to thicken to toothpaste consistency. If persistent diarrhoea remains a problem, the patient needs to be reviewed by their surgeon to identify the cause and receive appropriate treatment. Regular follow-up is recommended after J-pouch formation, and patients should count the number of bowel actions per day to establish a base line for improvement while their bowel is adjusting to a change of habit.

Figure 11.2 J-pouch surgery

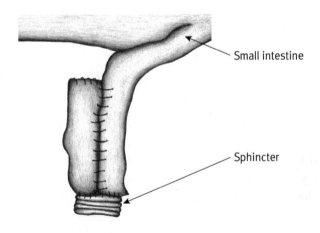

Small intestine

Sphincter

Figure 11.3 J-pouch fashioned out of small intestine

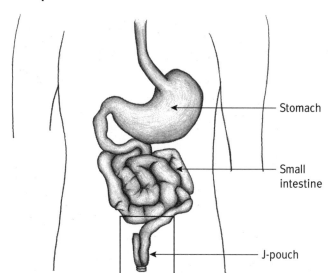

Stomach

Small
intestine

J-pouch

Managing your stoma

The key to managing your stoma is to be properly educated about
it and to surround yourself with supportive family and friends.
Major public hospitals have clinical nurse consultants, also called
stoma therapists. Before any surgery is planned, you should have a
pre-admission consultation with a stoma therapist. This meeting is
important for several reasons: to give you the counselling you may
need; to make sure you know what to expect from the surgery and
what's involved in the care of the stoma afterwards; and to work
out where the stoma will be positioned. You are usually encouraged to bring a friend or family member for support. Anything
that you haven't understood, or wanted to ask the surgeon on
previous occasions but didn't, can be discussed with the stoma
therapist. They will have pamphlets and booklets about your
procedure for you to take home so you will have more time to
understand what to expect.

After your surgery, the stoma therapist will work with you to make sure you can manage your stoma and will tell you when you are ready to go home. Most in-hospital education does not start until about day three after the operation. This is to give you time to recover from the procedure so that you are ready to learn about the care of the stoma. Then, over the next few days, the stoma therapist or an experienced nurse will teach you what you need to know, including lessons in appliance management.

Once you are out of hospital, you will be given regular follow-up appointments to check that you are managing and to answer any questions you may have. The first is usually one to two weeks after surgery. If for some reason, such as moving to a new area, you have not had contact with a stoma therapist, ask your GP to refer you to one, or ring your local hospital to get in touch with the stoma therapist who services your area. You can also ring the Australian Association of Stomal Therapy Nurses, or visit its website at www.stomaltherapy.com, to find a nurse in your area. It is a wonderful source of information, and, if you have any queries or doubts, talk to the association. In the meantime, here are some general principles on managing your stoma.

Skin care and hygiene

It is important to look after the peristomal skin. Check it regularly for irritation, either from the stick-on pouch, leakage, or body products and soaps. Make sure your pouch fits properly. Keep your stoma clean with soap and water. Do not use a dry face washer or other dry materials on the stoma as this can damage the mucosa. Dry the skin around the stoma thoroughly to ensure the pouch will stick. Avoid using creams or gels because these can affect the adhesion of the pouch. If you have any signs of skin redness or pain, contact your stoma therapist. You can shower and bath as you did before surgery, with or without the pouch on; whatever you prefer when you are at home. An ileostomy will continue to produce output while you are in the shower so leave your pouch on if you are using public baths. If your colostomy output is unpredictable, you should also keep the pouch on when showering away from home. Don't worry about water getting into the stoma. Also, wash your hands after handling your stoma or emptying your pouch. It is the same principle for anyone after using the toilet.

Odours

This is one of the concerns that bothers people most when faced with ostomy surgery. The technology of the pouches is excellent nowadays and they have an odour barrier inside the pouch to stop any odours getting out. The only time you should notice an odour is when the barrier is broken, such as when you are changing your pouch. For peace of mind, empty your ileostomy pouch when it is about one-third full: It will need to be emptied between four and six times in 24 hours. For a colostomy, change the pouch after a bowel action: typically, this is about one to three times a day. Some foods are prone to producing odorous stools. These are mentioned under dietary considerations later in this chapter.

Gas

Gas production in the bowel is normal. We all pass wind whether we admit it or not. It is no different when you have an ostomy. Gas will be produced and you may see your pouch expand. It comes from various sources including the foods you eat, swallowing air, chewing gum and drinking fizzy drinks. Some of the foods that increase gas production are listed under dietary considerations. Pouches with built-in filters should allow the gas to leave the pouch but without any noticeable odour.

Colonic irrigation

This is done to empty the bowel of faeces from the colostomy. It involves flushing out the bowel with warm water using a colostomy irrigation set. It needs to be taught by an experienced nurse and performed every one to two days. It is not widely done anymore. This is because it is time-consuming—it takes more than an hour—it can be an odorous procedure, and it is not as necessary because of the advanced easy-to-use pouches available today.

Stoma equipment

Figure 11.4 Ileostomy pouch

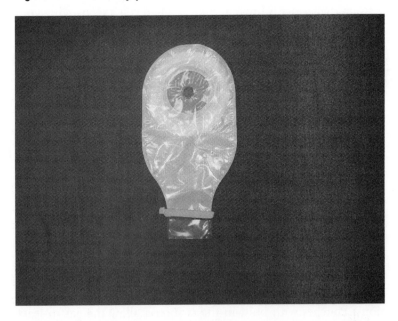

There are hundreds of stoma products on the market. Not all will be relevant to you. Ileostomies need drainable pouches that can be emptied into the toilet. This is quick and simple. After emptying the pouch, the end is resealed with a fold-up closure or clamp. The pouch is replaced every three days.

In contrast, colostomies need a closed pouch that is discarded after each bowel action. The pouch has an inbuilt filter to remove gas and odour. Without this, the pouch can expand and look odd underneath clothing.

Both types of pouches come in different materials, and your choice will depend on your needs. Some are see-through so that you can see the stoma and know when to change your bag; however, if you prefer not to see the contents, you can get an opaque pouch. Some are made of softer materials than others to provide comfort against the skin, and be cosmetically acceptable. Both systems come with pre-cut openings in the wafer and those that you have to cut yourself. Initially, you may want to cut the opening yourself as your stoma will change in size during the first six months after surgery. Once it has settled down, and if you have a stoma that is suitable, you can use pre-cut wafers to save time when changing bags. But, not everyone who has a stoma has a perfectly round shape and therefore pre-cut wafers may not be useful for them.

For people with a colostomy, there is also the option of a colostomy plug. This is a plug that is inserted into the stoma and expands to provide a good seal. These are very useful for people with regular bowel habits who work in physical jobs or play sport and do not want to worry about changing the pouch at work or during sporting activities. The plug also allows people with colostomies to be continent and odour and noise free. They are not suitable for everyone and you will need to do a familiarisation program over several weeks with an experienced stoma therapist to help you and your stoma get used to the plug before you use it regularly.

To help you navigate your way around the various products, talk to your stoma therapist. Some products come in two pieces: the bag and a flange. A flange is a plastic or rubber ring, or a ring that is incorporated into a wafer as part of a two-piece stoma appliance. Another term, often used when talking about stoma equipment is a skin barrier. A skin barrier describes the adhesive backing on any stoma appliance. Some products come with a belt that goes around your waist and attaches to the pouch to help you attain a good seal over the stoma. Sometimes the adhesive area of the pouch that goes over the stoma is curved. This is called convexity, and the idea of this design is to tilt the stoma forwards into the pouch so that it gets a better seal and is unlikely to leak. You may want to experiment with different types of pouches and convexities until you find the product that suits you best. Appliances with convexity are recommended for patients who have temporary loop ileostomies or retracted stomas. A retracted stoma is not ideal. It occurs when the stoma fails to protrude a few centimetres from the body as fashioned by the surgeon, and instead 'sinks' to be flush with the skin, or even dipping a little below. It is difficult to get a pouch to fit well over a retracted stoma, and it will require an experienced stoma therapist to help find the stoma products that will fit it best so that it is leak free.

Where to get stoma supplies?

There are about 35 000 Australians living with stomas. Thankfully, the federal government through the Australian Stoma Appliance Scheme provides stoma therapy appliances and products free of charge. Without this scheme, which began in the 1970s, many patients with stomas would have financial difficulties. The equipment is distributed by volunteers through stoma associations in each state (see the end of this chapter for details). You will need to become a member of a stoma association and have a Medicare card to be eligible to receive the free appliances.

Dietary considerations

The good news is that most medical professionals will tell you that you can have a normal diet once you are out of hospital and your stoma is functioning well. However, there are a few things to keep in mind, such as:

- Eat a healthy, well-balanced diet to keep up your nutrition and good health. The Australian diet is becoming one that is high in fat and low in fibre. Try to overcome this by making sure you get adequate fibre and minimise the fat in your diet. See chapter three for more information on healthy eating.

- Keep up your fluids, particularly if you have an ileostomy, as you will be losing more fluid than the average person because you are not getting reabsorption of water in the large bowel. It is recommended that you drink at least 2 litres of fluid a day. Drink more on hot days. Keep caffeine and alcohol to a minimum, as these can dehydrate you. People with colostomies can get constipation, so again it is advisable to keep up the fluids.

- Know which foods can increase gas production for you. The pouch technology has come a long way and filters are built into closed pouches to allow deodorised gas to escape. But, they are not always perfect. Foods that can increase gas production include: fizzy drinks, beer, dried peas or beans, onions, cabbage, broccoli, Brussels sprouts, cauliflower, milk and milk products, eggs, some spicy foods, baked beans and lentils. If you need fibre, this can increase gas production, so increase your fibre intake slowly over several weeks.

  People with an ileostomy need to thoroughly chew their food, particularly small, hard food like peanuts, and peas and fibrous vegetables, so that it does not cause a blockage.

- Some food can increase the stoma output, particularly for ileostomies. Different people will react to foods differently, but some foods and drinks that are known to increase output are: beans, beer, chocolate, caffeinated drinks, leafy green vegetables, raw fruit and vegetables, fresh fruit drinks, prunes and prune juice, and wholegrain cereals and bread.

- Some foods decrease output and thicken the waste. They include: ripe bananas, boiled white rice, noodles, cheese, peanut butter, mashed potatoes, white bread, pasta, yoghurt and apple sauce.
- Some foods can increase odour. These include: eggs, onions, spices, fish, asparagus, garlic, broccoli, cabbage, cauliflower and Brussels sprouts.
- Medications can affect the colour, odour and thickness of the faecal output. If you think this is happening to you, talk to your doctor or stoma therapist.

Complications

Once you have been home for a while, the stoma complications you need to watch out for include:

- Herniation—when the stoma prolapses and becomes large in size
- Skin problems around the stoma
- Stoma retraction—when the stoma sinks below the skin level
- Stenosis—a blocked or partially blocked stoma
- Granulomas—lumps on the stoma
- Stoma ulceration—when small ulcers appear on the mucosa
- Fistula formation—tracts around the stoma
- Bulges around the stoma.

Other general problems that may arise include:

- Dehydration—not drinking enough fluids
- Electrolyte imbalances—chemical imbalances that are usually a result of dehydration
- Bowel obstruction—blockage of the bowel.

If you experience any of these problems, see your doctor. Always seek immediate medical attention if your stoma changes colour, starts to bleed, or becomes painful or dries out.

Getting on with life with a stoma

Life with a stoma is no reason to stop doing things you enjoy. Here are some suggestions to make life with a stoma a little easier.

Clothes

Pouches are thin and will fit close to your body. You can tuck them into your underclothes or over the top, whatever you prefer. High-fitting underwear or Lycra sports shorts are sometimes worn to keep the pouch close to the body and disguised. Empty your ileostomy pouch when it is about one-third full so that it does not bulge under your clothes, and always empty colostomies after every bowel action. You should be able to wear almost any clothes you want. If you want to go swimming, choose a patterned swim-suit. Always empty your pouch before getting in the water. You can use waterproof tape to secure the edges of your skin barrier to make sure it stays in place, but it is unnecessary. Modern pouches should not smell or leak if they are well fitting.

Work and travel

Wait until your doctor says you are physically well enough before going back to work or travelling. Once you are ready, you should be able to do most things. If you have a job that involves travel or you want to take a vacation, plan ahead and pack your pouches in your carry-on luggage. Scissors are no longer allowed on aero-planes so remember to **cut your pouches or wafers to fit before you go if you do not use pre-cut bags.** Pack enough supplies to last the duration of your trip—it is a good idea to overestimate, so that you don't run out. It might be worth taking a travel certificate with you so that you don't have any problems when you go through customs in other countries. You can get this from your doctor. Always take your medications with you in case you cannot get them at your destination. Appliances should be stored in a cool place, away from heat and direct sunlight. To get the most use out of your equipment, use your older stock first.

If you have a very physical job and are fit enough to work, you may want to consider a plug if you have a colostomy. This makes it easier to move around without worrying about changing a pouch. If you have an ileostomy, make sure the pouch is securely tucked into your undergarments. Heat and perspiration can increase the wear and tear on your pouches. If required, see if there are more durable versions available to suit your occupation or the climate you live in or are travelling to.

Sport

You should be able to enjoy most sports other than extremely rough contact sports. Pouches are waterproof, so water sports are not a problem. If you like to jog and have an ileostomy, for your comfort and to avoid leaks get in the habit of emptying your pouch before you exercise and again once you are finished.

Sex

There is no physical reason not to be enjoying sex. But, understandably, it may take time for you to feel comfortable to be intimate with a partner. Ileostomy and colostomy surgery affects both people in a relationship. Your partner may be worried about hurting the stoma. You need to be open and honest with each other. Try and involve your partner in your education sessions about the stoma so that their fears can be allied. Women are usually still able to have children after stoma surgery and many men are still able to become fathers; however, surgery can result in impotence for men, particularly if the surgery involves the pelvis. If this is a problem for you, talk to your doctor, as there are options available including implants.

Before intimacy, make sure your pouch is empty. You can buy all types of appealing apparel to cover your pouch if you want to. If you have a colostomy, you may want to try a plug so that you needn't worry about skin-to-skin friction interfering with the pouch.

If you are in the early stages of dating and not sure about when to tell your date about your stoma, don't feel that you have to rush it. You will know when the timing is right for you. Anyone worth your attention will be understanding of your situation when you are ready to tell them. Understanding is the basis of all loving relationships, regardless of our health and lifestyle situations.

Some common questions about stomas

How often should I change my bag? I have an end ileostomy?

The manufacturers of the products recommend that a one-piece drainable bag can be worn for up to three days. Heat and moisture can shorten the life of a bag, so any physical exercise may cause more wear and tear. If you have a two-piece system with a wafer, the wafer may be worn for up to three days.

I have noticed some redness around the skin of my stoma and it is very sore. What should I do?

The skin around your stoma (the peristomal skin) should look just like the skin on your abdomen. To prevent skin irritation or other skin problems, you need a pouch that fits properly. Also, use commercial wipes sparingly. Instead use warm, soapy water, and a large cotton pad or cotton wool to wash around the skin. You need to check the skin each time you change your appliance. Swelling of the stoma, redness, rash or pain need to be investigated by your stoma therapist or doctor. They may be able to recommend a different type of pouching system.

I had surgery recently and have noticed my stoma has shrunk. Is this normal?

As you start to heal and the swelling from the surgery starts to subside, you will notice that your stoma will shrink a little. This is normal. The type of pouching system you used in the hospital will need to be reconsidered to allow for these changes. Talk to your stoma therapist about this; they will be able to tell you what pouch will best suit you now.

When should I tell my boyfriend that I have an ileostomy? We have only been going out for a few months?

This is a question that bothers many people living with a stoma. The answer depends on you. When will you feel comfortable talking about your stoma with your partner? You don't have to feel obligated to tell him that you have a stoma; it can wait until you feel ready. Most patients that have been through this say that they know within themselves when the time is right. If he is the caring partner that you expect, he will understand, but remember that it may be a shock for him, just as it was for you, and you need to allow time for him to come to terms with the news. Some partners are curious and he may have lots of questions. Make sure you are ready for these reactions.

After my shower when I am drying myself, my stoma bleeds. Is this okay?

The stoma is similar to the tissue found inside your cheek. It is mucosal tissue. This means it has lots of blood vessels close to the surface and if you rub it with something coarse, like a towel, it will bleed a little. It is not something to worry about, but try to avoid using rough and dry materials on the stoma. Dry the skin around the stoma, rather than worrying about the stoma itself. If you get excessive bleeding from the stoma, this is a different problem and you will need to see your doctor or contact your stoma therapist promptly.

Are there foods I need to avoid after having an ileostomy?

You should eat normally. Just remember to chew, chew, chew. You can make a note of the effect of each food on the output of your stoma. Ileostomy output is like toothpaste so you will need to keep your fluids up to ensure that you don't become dehydrated. Aim for 2 litres a day and more in hot weather. Always chew your food well. Some small hard foods like nuts and fibrous vegetables can cause blockages—so be **wary** of these, and thoroughly chew all food.

Further information

Stoma associations and related organisations

The Australian Council of Stoma Associations (ACSA) is the umbrella group for the 22 regional stoma associations in Australia. For information on getting free stoma supplies, to find your local association, or for more information on living with a stoma visit: www.australianstoma.com.au.

The Australian Association of Stomal Therapy Nurses Inc. will help find a stoma therapist in your area; go to the website: www. stomaltherapy.com.

District nursing services operate in most areas of Australia and some have experienced stoma therapists who can help you manage your stoma at home if you need more help. Ring your local hospital or doctor for the nearest centre. Victoria has a state-based service: www.rdns.com.au/Services/Stomal+therapy.htm.

The Federation of New Zealand Ostomy Societies, Inc. is an umbrella organisation that serves the needs of New Zealanders with stomas. It is estimated that 5000 New Zealanders have a stoma. For more details, visit: www.ostomyinternational.org/new zealand.html.

Stoma support groups

YOU (Young Ostomates United) is an Australian-based support group for young people with stomas and is located in Melbourne. It organises events and provides members with support and regular newsletters. Visit the group online at: http://home.vicnet. net.au/~youinc/. Or contact them at:

Young Ostomates United Inc.
PO Box 1433 MDC
Narre Warren Vic. 3805
Australia

OST WEST Support Group is a Victorian support group based in Melton for people who have had ostomy surgery.
Contact: Patricia Young (founder)
Phone: (03) 9743 5868
Website: http://mc2.vicnet.net.au/home/ostwest/index.html

Australian Crohn's and Colitis Association (ACCA) is a not-for-profit membership group that provides up-to-date information on IBD and support for members.

Australian Crohn's and Colitis Association (ACCA)
Level 1, 462 Burwood Road
Hawthorn, Vic. 3122
Phone: (03) 9815 1266
Website: www.acca.net.au
Email: info@acca.net.au

Or, contact the ACCA office in your state:
New South Wales   Phone: 1800 220 522
Northern Territory   Phone: 1800 220 522
Queensland   Phone: 1800 220 522
South Australia   Phone: (08) 8449 4357
Tasmania   Phone: (03) 6437 6184
Victoria   Phone: (03) 9726 9008
Western Australia   Phone: 1800 138 029

Nidkids, the Australian neuronal intestinal dysplasia support group, is dedicated to helping children with NID, and their families. NID is a congenital condition involving an abnormal nerve supply to the bowel causing bowel problems.
PO Box 30
Lilydale, Vic. 3140
Phone: (03) 9727 2997
Fax: (03) 9727 4632
Email: mail@nidkids.org.au
Website: www.nidkids.org.au

Books

Managing Your Colostomy: Patient education series
A useful book provided free of charge by your stoma therapist. It goes through the basics of colostomy care and is produced by the stoma appliance manufacturer Hollister. For more information, phone FreeCall 1800 335 911.

Managing Your Ileostomy: Patient education series and *Managing Your Loop Ileostomy: Patient education series*
These useful books are provided free of charge by your stoma therapist. They go into details of ileostomy care. They are easy to understand and are up to date. They are produced by Hollister. For more information, phone FreeCall 1800 335 911.

Useful websites

The Gut Foundation provides public education and promotes research into digestive disorders to improve gastrointestinal health: www.gut.nsw.edu.au.

The International Ostomy Association is committed to the improvement of the quality of life of ostomates and those with related surgeries, worldwide: www.ostomyinternational.org.

The various pouch manufacturers are obviously commercial but they do have some helpful general advice about stoma care. Websites include: www.dansac.com.au and www.hollister.com.au.

An American not-for-profit chat and information website about J-pouch surgery and temporary stomas has qualified registered nurses available to answer questions: www.j-pouch.org.

Other national ostomy associations include:
United Ostomy Associations of America (USA): www. uoaa.org
The Ileostomy Association of UK: www.the-ia.org.uk
British Colostomy Association: www.bcass.org.uk
United Ostomy Association of Canada: www.ostomy canada.ca

A final word . . .

One of the reasons that I chose to study gastrointestinal medicine is because the outlook for many people's health is positive. Certainly patients are diagnosed with chronic illnesses that cannot be cured, such as Crohn's disease and coeliac disease, but even then, the quality of life that most people can live when they have experienced and competent health management is usually good. From a doctor's perspective, even the most difficult cases usually have more than one treatment option and it is very satisfying when you are able to see someone's health improve, enabling them to get on with living and not simply surviving.

Also, each year across the globe, governments, private companies and research institutes are investing hundreds of millions of dollars to further research the gastrointestinal diseases discussed here, and to develop new drugs and treatments. For example, irritable bowel syndrome has become an increasingly well-recognised condition and subsequently better understood. Major advances in the knowledge of the possible underlying mechanisms causing the disease have led to the development of a number of specific drugs aimed at addressing these. Tegaserod, a drug that acts on the nervous system in the bowel, has been shown to be very effective, at least in the short term, for constipation-predominant IBS (IBS-C). Its long-term benefits will be known as time progresses. Similar drugs have been developed for diarrhoea-predominant IBS (IBS-D) that showed great promise, but were withdrawn because of potential side effects. Current developments are focused on these types of drugs. In the area of diet, there is no doubt that dietary manipulation has been under done in IBS, and the value of FODMAP and fructose intolerance is an exciting new area of interest.

With respect to ulcer disease, the good news is that *Helicobacter pylori* is becoming less common with widespread use of antibiotics and better living conditions throughout the world. However, less fortunate has been the recent international scandal regarding potential heart problems associated with the newer anti-inflammatory drugs, which has led to an increasing reliance on older drugs that are well known to cause peptic ulcers. This is not likely to be resolved anytime soon, meaning that there will be increased reliance on preventative use of other drugs such as PPIs in combating peptic ulcer disease.

Turning to coeliac disease, there is no doubt that it also has been under recognised by the medical community worldwide, and particularly in the United States, until more recently. Great advances have been made into the understanding of the cause of coeliac disease, and possible vaccines to prevent it. This advancement, along with the development of genetically modified grains that do not contain gluten, is probably about five to ten years away from release. As coeliac disease becomes more well-recognised, there will be a greater proportion of people diagnosed after very mild or even asymptomatic disease. The importance of strict dietary control in this group is yet to be seen. Overall, the future looks more promising for coeliac sufferers.

As for the management and treatment of inflammatory bowel disease, they are being based around the benefits drawn from the translation of molecular biology into clinical medicine. For example, biological therapies created in the laboratory to combat the immune system when it malfunctions are revolutionising the management of IBD and are expected to continue to do so. As the genetic component of IBD becomes better understood, it is probable that IBD will be seen as a group of similar but unique diseases, all with specific treatments. Further, the technology available today can help predict which treatments are more likely to be effective, and which ones are likely to cause a side effect, in any particular person through genetic analysis (pharmaco-genomics). On the dietary front, probiotics are in vogue and are likely to continue to be a popular way of treating problems in the gut. It is expected that 'designer probiotics' will be tailored to different problems, particularly in IBD.

Lastly, we hope this book has lifted some of the myths and misconceptions about the GIT and its function, and given some insight into the best ways to manage your illness, diet and lifestyle to prevent further episodes. Most importantly, we hope this book helps you to improve your digestive health and to enjoy life's wonderful pleasures of eating, drinking and socialising.

Andrew Brett, 2007

Further resources

Throughout this book every effort has been made to help you find the best information available about gastrointestinal problems and their treatments by including the latest addresses, telephone numbers and websites of organisations, support groups, government agencies and others. We are living in a global age and access to information is not limited to your physical location, so for this reason many overseas organisations have been listed at the end of chapters if their information is thought to be accurate and reflective of the advice given in Australia and New Zealand. In this section of the book, the information will be limited to resources in Australia and New Zealand so that more of these can be listed at a local level. Sometimes Internet, telephone and address details can change as organisations move, close or merge, and we apologise in advance for any difficulty in finding recommended information in the event this has occurred since the time of publication. Finally, all information is provided free of any commercial interest or relationship. All information in this book, including drug names, is provided independent of any influence or motive other than to give you knowledge so that your health might benefit.

Alternative therapies

Australian College of Natural Medicine
Website: www.acnm.edu.au

Queensland
362 Water Street
Fortitude Valley Qld 4006
Phone: (07) 3257 1883
Fax: (07) 3257 1889

1 Nerang Street
Southport Qld 4215
Phone: (07) 5503 0977
Fax: (07) 5503 0988

Victoria
368 Elizabeth Street
Melbourne Vic. 3000
Phone: (03) 9662 9911
Fax: (03) 9662 9414

2A Cambridge Street
Box Hill Vic. 3128
Phone: (03) 9890 5599
Fax: (03) 9898 8260

Western Australia
170 Wellington Street
East Perth WA 6004
Phone: (08) 9225 2900
Fax: (08) 9225 2999

This is a commercial telephone and web directory for therapists across Australia: www.naturaltherapypages.com.au.

This is another useful directory with a listing of schools and colleges and therapists: www.austherapy.com.au.

Continence

The Continence Foundation of Australia (CFA) was established in 1989 to help the estimated two million Australians with urinary and/or faecal incontinence. Contact the national office:

AMA House
293 Royal Parade
Parkville Vic. 3052
Phone: (03) 9347 2522
Helpline (FreeCall): 1800 330 066
Fax: (03) 9347 2533
Email: info@continence.org.au
Website: www.contfound.org.au

New Zealand Continence Association Inc. (NZCA) is a continence organisation providing answers to questions, and downloadable information sheets on male and female continence issues and bowel control.
Jan Zander
Executive Officer
PO Box 270
Drury 1730 NZ
Email: jan@continence.org.nz
Website: www.continence.org.nz

Diet and nutrition

Find a dietitian in your state or territory by contacting the **Dietitians Association of Australia**. This site also has useful dietary tips and advice: www.daa.asn.au.

For tips on eating healthily and adding fibre to your diet: www.betterhealth.vic.gov.au.

Nutrition Australia is a not-for-profit, non-government, community-based organisation that aims to educate the population about healthy eating and living: www.nutritionaustralia.org.

For vegetarian dietary options, contact the **Vegetarian Society** at: www.vegsoc.org/info/gluten.html.

Drugs

The National Prescribing Service is funded by the Australian federal government's Department of Health and Ageing, and is incorporated as a limited company with a membership of prominent health, medical and consumer organisations. It provides booklets and online information about your drugs and how to use medicines safely.

PO Box 1147
Strawberry Hills NSW 2012
Phone: (02) 8217 8700
Phone: 1300 888 763
Fax: (02) 9211 7578
Email: info@nps.org.au
Website: www.nps.org.au

The National Preferred Medicines Centre Inc. (PreMeC) was set up by a group of New Zealand doctors from varied medical disciplines with the aim of improving prescribing habits and the safe use of medicines.

Email: info@premec.org.nz

Website: www.medimate.org.au

Government health websites

HealthInsite is a website to provide information about varied health topics from health organisations, government agencies, and educational and research institutions: www.healthin site.gov.au.

The National Public Toilet map is found on a website funded by the federal government that locates public toilet facilities in Australian cities, towns, rural areas, and along major travel routes: www. toiletmap.gov.au.

Journals

The *Medical Journal of Australia* website has some good articles on peptic ulcer disease. This site is better suited to health professionals who are familiar with medical language: www.mja.com.au.

The *New Zealand Medical Journal* is available online. It is designed for health professionals and has a user-friendly searchable database: www.nzma.org.nz/journal/index.shtml.

The Australian Coeliac is produced four times a year. It is available to members of the Australian Coeliac Society and gives members information, updates, members' stories, new recipes and food ideas, travel information, and upcoming events and activities. Visit the website: www.coeliac.org.au/the-australian-coeliac.htm.

The *Ostomy Australia Magazine* is available online at www.australianstoma.com.au/publications.htm.

Medical organisations

Gastroenterological Society of Australia (GESA)
145 Macquarie Street
Sydney NSW 2000
Phone: (02) 9256 5454
Fax: (02) 9241 4586
Email: gesa@gesa.org.au
Website: www.gesa.org.au

The Gut Foundation is an Australian organisation that provides professional and public education, and promotes research into digestive disorders to improve gastrointestinal health.
c/- Gastrointestinal Unit
The Prince of Wales Hospital
Randwick NSW 2031
Phone: (02) 9382 2749
Fax: (02) 9382 2828
Email: gutfound@gut.nsw.edu.au
Website: www.gut.nsw.edu.au

The New Zealand Society of Gastroenterology is the national organisation of gastroenterologists. The website has little information but, for patients, there is still a useful resource list about gastrointestinal conditions: www.nzsg.org.nz.

This online information service set up by Australian gastro-enterologists and health professionals includes dietary information for IBS and other digestive disorders: www.gastro.net.au.

The Colorectal Surgical Society of Australia and New Zealand was formed by a group of surgeons to speak about all matters relating to colorectal surgery. The website has excellent information about many GIT diseases.
Level 2, 4 Cato Street
Hawthorn Vic. 3122
Phone: (03) 9822 8522
Fax: (03) 9822 8400
Email: secretariat@cssanz.org
Website: www.cssa.org.au

The National Health & Medical Research Council has information for the prevention, early detection and management of colorectal cancer, and a guide for patients and their families: www.nhmrc.health.gov.au.

Stoma information

There are an estimated 35 000 Australians living with stomas. **The Australian Council of Stoma Associations (ACSA)** is the umbrella group for the 22 regional stoma associations in Australia. For information on getting free stoma supplies, to find your local association, or for more information on living with a stoma, visit: www.australianstoma.com.au.

Australian Capital Territory
ACT & District Stoma Association   (02) 6205 1055

New South Wales
Colostomy Association   (02) 9656 4315
Ileostomy Association   (02) 9568 2799

Northern Territory

Cancer Council of the Northern Territory	(08) 8927 6389
FreeCall	1800 678 123

Queensland

Gold Coast Ostomy Association	(07) 5594 7633
North Queensland Ostomy Association	(07) 4775 2303
Queensland Colostomy Association	(07) 3848 7178
Queensland Stoma Association	(07) 3359 7570
Toowoomba & South West Ostomy Association	(07) 4636 9701
Wide Bay Ostomy Association	(07) 4150 2074

South Australia

Colostomy Association	(08) 8354 2618
Ileostomy Association	(08) 8234 2678

Tasmania

Ileostomy & Colostomy Association	(03) 6223 2974

Victoria

Bendigo & District Ostomy Association	(03) 5441 7520
Colostomy Association	(03) 9650 1666
Geelong Ostomy Association	(03) 5222 3168
Ileostomy Association	(03) 9650 9040
Ostomy Association of Melbourne	(03) 9508 1879
Peninsula Ostomy Association	(03) 9783 6473
Victorian Children's Ostomy Association	(03) 9345 5325
Warrnambool & District Ostomy Association	(03) 5563 1446

Western Australia

West Australian Ostomy Association	(08) 9272 1833

To find a stoma therapist in your area, visit the **Australian Association of Stomal Therapy Nurses Inc.** website: www.stomal therapy.com.

Federation of New Zealand Ostomy Societies, Inc. (FNZOS) is an umbrella organisation that serves the needs of New Zealanders with stoma. It is estimated that 5000 New Zealanders have a stoma.
Mrs Robyn Tourell (secretary)
Phone: (03) 454 5330
Email: tourell.r@xtra.co.nz
Website: www.ostomyinternational.org/newzealand.html

The pouch manufacturers are obviously commercial enterprises but they do have useful information on their websites about stoma care:
www.dansac.com.au
www.coloplast.com
www.coloplast.com.au
www.hollister.com.au

Stomal support groups

OST WEST Support Group is an Australian support group based in Melton, Victoria. It is for people who have had stoma surgery.
Contact: Patricia Young (founder)
Phone: (03) 9743 5868
Website: http://mc2.vicnet.net.au/home/ostwest/index.html

YOU (Young Ostomates United) is an Australian support group, based in Melbourne, dedicated to young people with stomas. It organises events, and provides members with support and regular newsletters.

Young Ostomates United Inc.
PO Box 1433 MDC
Narre Warren Vic. 3805
Website: http://home.vicnet.net.au/~youinc

Support and self-help groups

The Cancer Council Australia is Australia's national non-government cancer control organisation. It funds cancer research and provides information and support for people affected by cancer.
GPO Box 4708, Sydney NSW 2001
Level 5, Medical Foundation Building
92–94 Parramatta Road
Camperdown NSW 2050
Phone: (02) 9036 3100
Fax: (02) 9036 3101
Email: info@cancer.org.au
Website: www.cancer.org.au

Children and bowel problems

Nidkids is an Australian neuronal intestinal dysplasia support group dedicated to helping children with NID, and their families. NID is a congenital condition involving an abnormal nerve supply to the bowel causing bowel problems.
PO Box 30
Lilydale Vic. 3140
Phone: (03) 9727 2997
Fax: (03) 9727 4632
Email: mail@nidkids.org.au
Website: www.nidkids.org.au

Chronic illness

Chronic Illness Alliance Vic. (CIA) has 39 member organisations across Australia. It aims to improve health policy and health services for all people with chronic illnesses and provides regular newsletters for its members.
818 Burke Road
Camberwell Vic. 3124
Phone: (03) 9805 9126
Email: mail@chronicillness.org.au
Website: www.chronicillness.org.au

Coeliac disease

The Coeliac Society of Australia
PO Box 703
Chatswood NSW 2057
Phone: (02) 9411 4100
Fax: (02) 9413 1296
Website: www.coeliac.org.au

New South Wales
PO Box 703
Chatswood NSW 2057
Phone: (02) 9411 4100
Fax: (02) 9413 1296
Website: www.nswcoeliac.org.au

Victoria
PO Box 89, Holmesglen Vic. 3148
11 Barlyn Road
Mt Waverley Vic. 3149

Phone: (03) 9808 5566
Fax: (03) 9808 9922
FreeCall: 1300 458 836
Website: www.vic.coeliac.org.au

Queensland
PO Box 2110, Fortitude Valley BC 4006
Level 1, Local Government House
25 Evelyn Street
Newstead Qld 4006
Phone: (07) 3854 0123
Fax: (07) 3854 0121
Website: http://qld.coeliac.org.au

South Australia
Unit 5, 88 Glynburn Road
Hectorville SA 5073
Phone: (08) 8365 1488 or (08) 8336 1476
Fax: (08) 8365 1265
Website: http://sa.coeliac.org.au

Western Australia
PO Box 1344, East Victoria Park WA 6981
931 Albany Highway
East Victoria Park WA 6101
Phone: (08) 9470 4122
Fax: (08) 9470 4166
FreeCall: 1300 458 836
Website: www.wa.coeliac.org.au

Tasmania
PO Box 159
Launceston Tas. 7250
Phone: (03) 6427 2844
Fax: (03) 6344 4284
Website: http://tas.coeliac.org.au

Northern Territory
The Coeliac Society of Australia
PO Box 703
Chatswood NSW 2057
Phone: (02) 9411 4100
Fax: (02) 9413 1296
Website: www.coeliac.org.au

Coeliac Society of New Zealand Inc.
PO Box 35 724
Browns Bay 1330
Auckland
Phone: +64 (09) 820 5157
Fax: +64 (09) 820 5187
Website: www.colourcards.com/coeliac/

IBD

Australian Crohn's and Colitis Association (ACCA)
Level 1, 462 Burwood Rd
Hawthorn Vic 3122
Phone: (03) 9815 1266
Email: info@acca.net.au
Website: www.acce.net.au

Or, contact the office in your state:

New South Wales	Phone: 1800 220 522
Northern Territory	Phone: 1800 220 522
Queensland	Phone: 1800 220 522
South Australia	Phone: (08) 8449 4357
Tasmania	Phone: (03) 6437 6184
Victoria	Phone: (03) 9726 9008
Western Australia	Phone: 1800 138 029

IBS

Irritable Bowel Information & Support Association of Australia (IBIS Australia)
PO Box 7092
Sippy Downs Qld 5456
Phone: (07) 3907 0527
Email: contact@ibis-australia.org
Website: www.ibis-australia.org

Reflux

A New Zealand website, sponsored by the **Gastric Reflux Support Network New Zealand for Parents of Infants and Children Charitable Trust (GRSNNZ)**, provides information to parents who have children that suffer from reflux: www.crying overspiltmilk.co.nz.

GESA has some useful information on its website about reflux: www.gesa.org.au/leaflets/heartburn.cfm.

Quit smoking

Quitline
Phone: 13 7848 in Australia
Website: www.quit.org.au

Recipes

This book has talked about the important role that diet plays in the management of many gastrointestinal tract problems. This is particularly the case with the management of diverticulitis, haemorrhoids, irritable bowel syndrome, lactose intolerance and coeliac disease. To address the food requirements of these GIT problems, some popular recipes are included here to get you started on tasty, healthy eating to improve your gastrointestinal health.

Recipes high in fibre

If you have diverticulitis or haemorrhoids, a high-fibre diet is central to managing your illness. A high-fibre diet is also thought to help prevent the development of bowel cancer and is particularly recommended for people with a family history of the disease.

In many people with constipation-dominant IBS, a high-fibre diet can also be beneficial; although this is not the case for everyone, it is worth a trial. If a high-fibre diet doesn't work for you in controlling your IBS, then a low-irritant diet, *without* fructose or other FODMAPs, may be more suitable (see recipes below). To understand your dietary needs best, it is recommended you have the guidance of a dietitian experienced in managing IBS.

Garden pea soup

1 onion, diced
3 sticks celery, chopped
2 potatoes, peeled and diced
1 tablespoon butter
1 bay leaf
1 sprig of thyme
2 litres chicken stock
750 g garden peas (fresh or frozen)
salt and white pepper to taste
sour cream, to garnish

Sweat onion, celery and potato in butter with herbs in a soup saucepan over a medium heat. Add stock and simmer for 15 minutes. Add peas and boil for a further 3 minutes, then blend. Season with salt and white pepper. Garnish with sour cream. Serves 6.

Vietnamese chicken salad with noodles

Dressing:
2 cloves garlic, finely chopped
juice of 3 limes
3 tablespoons fish sauce
2 tablespoons brown sugar
2 teaspoons peanut oil (or vegetable oil)
1 tablespoon rice vinegar
1 chilli, seeded and chopped

200 g rice noodles

Salad:
2 cooked, skinned chicken breasts, thinly sliced
1 cup grated carrot
1 cup shredded mint leaves
handful of fresh coriander, to garnish
½ cup roasted peanuts, to garnish

Combine all dressing ingredients and leave for half an hour. Pour boiling water over the rice noodles and leave for 3 minutes, then strain. Combine all salad ingredients and toss through with noodles and dressing. Garnish with coriander and peanuts. Serves 4.

Rice pudding

butter
2 eggs
2 cups milk
2 tablespoons sugar
1 teaspoon vanilla essence
30 ml brandy (optional)
4 tablespoons short-grain brown rice, washed
sprinkle or slice of nutmeg

Preheat oven to 160° Celsius and butter a 750 ml pie dish. Lightly beat eggs with milk and sugar. Then stir in vanilla essence and brandy if using. Put rice in dish and pour over the liquid ingredients. Bake for 90 minutes, then sprinkle or grate nutmeg on top and serve. Serves 4.

Vitality cake

3 very ripe bananas
1 cup wholemeal flour
1 cup soy flour
1 cup wheat germ
1 cup All-bran
½ cup sultanas
1 cup dried apples
1 cup dates, pitted
1 tablespoon sesame seeds
1 tablespoon desiccated coconut
1½ cups milk

Mash bananas. Preheat oven to 180° Celsius. Combine bananas with the rest of the ingredients and bake in a loaf tin for 45 minutes.

Gluten-free and low-irritant recipes

If you have coeliac disease, it is paramount that you remove gluten, found in most wheat products, from your diet. The recipes below are suitable for people with coeliac disease. The recipes are also lactose free and fructose free (unless otherwise stated) and may benefit some people with IBS, lactose intolerance and fructose intolerance. Some of these recipes (marked with *) were provided from the cookbook, *Irresistibles for the Irritable*, written by Sue Shepherd, an experienced Australian dietitian specialising in coeliac and GIT diseases. Sue's PhD research focuses on fructose intolerance.

Mini frittatas

1 clove garlic
25 g butter or margarine
1 onion
100 g baby spinach, chopped
4 eggs
60g Parmesan cheese
100 g semi-dried tomatoes or 1 tomato, sliced
basil leaves (optional)

Crush garlic in the butter until soft. Chop the onion and sauté in the butter. Let cool. Cook the spinach for 2 minutes in the microwave on medium–high. Let cool.

Lightly beat the eggs, then add the spinach, onion and Parmesan.

Preheat oven to 180° Celsius. Grease 12 mini muffin tins or small, shallow cake tins. Spoon a small amount of egg mixture into each one until half-full and top with a couple of pieces of tomato.

Bake for 8–10 minutes or until the frittatas are set. Slide knife around each to loosen and turn out.

Decorate with basil leaves if desired.

Lemon risotto

1 lemon
300 ml dry white wine
1½ litres chicken stock
120 g unsalted butter
1 small onion, very finely chopped
600 g arborio rice
90 g grated Parmesan cheese
3 tablespoons finely chopped parsley
cracked pepper

Remove zest from lemon and reserve. Heat the wine and stock in a saucepan over medium heat.

While this is heating, use a heavy-based deep frying pan to melt 60 g of the butter, gently, and sauté onion. Add the rice and increase the heat (not too hot). Stir constantly to coat rice with butter. Add 1 cup of hot stock and stir. Simmer, keep stirring, and add 1 cup hot stock at a time until liquid is absorbed; don't drown the rice. After about 20 minutes, check rice is cooked by tasting: rice grains should be firm but tender. When rice is ready, stir in cheese, remaining half of the butter, parsley and lemon zest. Cover for 2 minutes and sprinkle with pepper to serve. Serves 6.

Penne with meatballs

1 kg lean minced beef
1 cup (220 g) cooked long-grain rice
90 g Parmesan cheese, grated
1 egg, beaten
2 cloves garlic, crushed
4 tablespoons fresh basil, chopped
¼ cup fresh parsley, chopped
½ teaspoon cayenne pepper
salt and freshly ground black pepper to taste
2 cups (500 ml) puréed tomato
¼ cup fresh basil, chopped, extra
500 g gluten-free penne pasta, cooked
additional Parmesan cheese, if desired

Combine mince, cooked rice, cheese, egg, garlic, basil, parsley, cayenne pepper, salt and pepper in a large mixing bowl. Shape into golfball-size balls and cook in a large non-stick frying pan over medium heat until browned and cooked through. Pour puréed tomato over meatballs, and add extra basil. Cook, simmering, for 2–3 minutes. Spoon meatballs and sauce over cooked pasta, and top with Parmesan cheese if desired. Serves 4.

*Berry friands

140 g unsalted butter
2 cups (280 g) pure icing sugar, plus extra to dust
¼ cup (40 g) gluten-free cornflour
¼ cup (45 g) rice flour
1¼ cups (125 g) almond meal
5 egg whites, lightly whisked
1 tablespoon lemon juice
2 teaspoons vanilla essence
150 g blueberries, boysenberries or raspberries

Preheat oven to 180° Celsius. Lightly grease 12 friand pans. Melt butter in a small saucepan over low heat. Heat for 3–4 minutes until flecks of brown appear. Set aside. Sift icing sugar and flours three times into a bowl. Mix in almond meal, combining well. Add egg whites, lemon juice, vanilla and butter to dry ingredients. Use a metal spoon to combine.

Spoon mixture into prepared pans until they are two-thirds full. Add berries, centred on top of batter. Bake in preheated oven for 12–15 minutes until light golden and firm to touch (a skewer inserted into the centre should come out clean). Allow to stand for 5 minutes before removing from tins, then place on wire rack to cool. Dust with pure icing sugar before serving. Makes 12.

*Blackberry white chocolate cheesecake

1 × 200 g packet plain gluten-free sweet biscuits
60 g butter, melted
410 g canned blackberries, drained, reserve I tablespoon liquid
½ cup (125 ml) boiling water
1 tablespoon gelatine
150 g white chocolate
500 g reduced-fat cream cheese
1 × 400 g can of sweetened condensed skim milk
2 teaspoons vanilla essence

Crush biscuits to form fine crumbs. Add melted butter and mix until well combined. Press evenly into the base of a 19-cm spring-form tin. Scatter tinned blackberries over biscuit base, ensuring it is evenly covered. Set aside.

Combine boiling water and gelatine in a small heatproof bowl. Set bowl over larger bowl of boiling water, stirring constantly until all gelatine is dissolved. Melt white chocolate in a bowl set over a small saucepan of simmering water. Stir to ensure it is completely melted. In a food processor, combine cream cheese, sweetened condensed milk, vanilla essence, dissolved gelatine and melted chocolate. Blend until well combined and even in consistency, then pour filling mixture over prepared base. Splash drops of reserved blackberry liquid on top of cheesecake. Run a knife or skewer in a straight motion up and down through drops, to form streaks on top of the cheesecake. Refrigerate for 3–4 hours or until set. Serves 10.

*Note: For the lactose intolerant, this dessert is unsuitable. Half-serves may be tolerated.

Shortbread

2⅓ cups (275 g) maize flour
1 cup (125 g) pure icing sugar
⅓ cup (50 g) soya flour
¼ cup (25 g) rice flour
250 g butter, at room temperature
caster or vanilla sugar (optional)

Preheat oven to 150° Celsius. Sift together the dry ingredients. Rub in butter with dry ingredients until it forms a dough. Roll the dough between two sheets of waxed paper to about 1.25 cm thickness. Peel off the top layer of paper and cut the dough into pieces about 2.5 × 7.5 cm. Lift pieces off the paper and place on a baking sheet, allowing room for spreading. Bake until faintly tinged golden around the edges, about 45 minutes. The shortbread can be sprinkled with caster sugar or vanilla sugar 10 minutes before the end of baking. Allow to cool, and store in an airtight container. Makes about 36 pieces.

Glossary

Abscess Localised accumulation of pus.

Absorption When food nutrients move from the intestine into the bloodstream.

Acid brash Sensation of acid coming up into one's mouth.

Acute Occurring suddenly or needing immediate medical attention.

Adenocarcinoma A malignant growth of glandular tissue.

Aerophagia The habit of swallowing air.

Allergen Something that triggers an allergic reaction.

Anaemia A decrease in the number of circulating red blood cells and/or the amount of haemoglobin in the blood.

Analgesia Pain-relieving medication.

Aperient Medication to treat constipation.

Bile Yellowish-green slimy fluid made by the gall bladder to help break down fats in the process of digestion.

Chyme The name given to churned food matter in the digestive system.

Coeliac disease Medical condition caused by gluten intolerance; called also coeliac sprue, gluten-sensitive enteropathy, non-tropical sprue or sprue.

Colic Cramp-like pain.

Colitis Inflammation of the large intestine.

Colon Large bowel, also called large intestine.

Colonoscopy A medical instrument that examines the colon.

Colostomy A surgically created opening on the abdominal skin to allow faeces to be expelled from the colon.

Crohn's disease An inflammatory bowel disease that can affect any part of the GIT.

Diaphragm Large band of muscle that sits under the ribs and aids breathing.

Digestion The physical breakdown of food into smaller particles in the stomach.

Diverticula More than one diverticulum.

Diverticulitis Inflammation of diverticula.

Diverticulum A small finger-like outpouching of the bowel wall.

Docosahexaenoic acid (DHA) An omega-3 polyunsaturated fatty acid found in fish.

Duodenum The first part of the small intestine.

Dyspepsia Abdominal pain; stomach upset.

Dysphagia Difficulty in swallowing.

Eicosapentaenoic acid (EPA) An omega-3 polyunsaturated fatty acid found in fish.

Elemental diet A liquid diet that does not need to be broken down by the small intestine.

Emetic A substance that causes vomiting.

Enzymes Chemical substances produced by the body to help digest food.

Fibromyalgia A disorder that causes muscle pain and fatigue.

Fistula Abnormal passage between two organs or between an organ and a cavity or the exterior, i.e. skin.

Flatus Gas produced in the bowel.

FODMAPs An acronym to describe five food elements. It stands for fermentable oligo-, di- and mono-saccharides and polyols.

Fructans A type of dietary fibre, includes inulin and oliogofructose.

Fructose A sugar or short-chained carbohydrate found naturally in fruit.

Gall bladder A pear-shaped organ that stores bile.

Gastroenteritis An acute infection of the bowel.

Gastrointestinal system (GIT) This is where digestion and absorption of nutrients occurs; it is a 7–8 metre continuous pipe that extends from the mouth to the anus.

Gluten A substance found in some cereals, especially wheat.

Glycaemic index (GI) The measurement of how a carbohydrate food affects glucose levels in the blood, in particular the rate of absorption of carbohydrate.

Haemorrhage Bleeding.

Haemorrhoids This usually refers to a prolapse of the anal cushions in the rectum.

Halitosis Bad breath.

Heartburn Burning pain that occurs after eating, usually caused by reflux; indigestion.

Helicobacter pylori (H. pylori) A bacterium in the stomach that causes peptic ulcers.

Hiatus hernia A protrusion of the stomach through the oesophageal opening of the diaphragm.

Ileostomy A surgically created opening connecting the ileum to the abdominal wall to allow faeces to be expelled.

Ileum The last section of small intestine before it joins the large intestine.

Ileus Cessation of peristalsis of the bowel.

Inflammatory bowel disease (IBD) Refers to ulcerative colitis and Crohn's disease.

Irritable bowel syndrome (IBS) Hypersensitive bowel condition that causes diarrhoea and constipation.

Ischaemia Restricted blood flow causing tissue death.

Jaundice Yellow colour in the skin, the mucous membranes or the eyes.

Jejunum Section of the small intestine.

Lactase Enzyme that breaks down lactose.

Lactose Sugar found in milk.

Large intestine The colon or large bowel.

Liver Large boomerang-shaped organ on the upper right side of the body below the diaphragm, with many functions including metabolising carbohydrates.

Lower oesophageal sphincter (LOS) A sphincter that prevents backflow of stomach contents into the oesophagus.

Malabsorption The failure of nutrients to be absorbed properly in the intestine.

Mucous membrane Tissue that secretes and is protected by mucous.

Nausea The feeling of wanting to vomit.

Nutrient A basic food component: carbohydrate, fat, protein. Micronutrients include vitamins, minerals and salt.

Obstruction A blockage.

Odynophagia Pain on swallowing.

Oesophagus Also called the gullet, the tube connecting the mouth to the stomach.

Osteoporosis Disease of bone degeneration caused by lack of calcium in the bones.

Ostomy Another term for stoma.

Parietal The outside layer of the membrane lining the peritoneum.

Pathogen A living substance that causes disease or illness in its host.

Perforation A hole; in the GIT, a perforation can cause abdominal contents to leak into the peritoneal cavity.

Peristalsis The wave-like motion caused by muscles inside the GIT that moves food through the tract from the mouth to the anus.

Peritonitis Inflammation of the peritoneal membrane.

Peritoneum The membrane which lines the abdominal cavity.

Pharynx The throat.

Polyp A tumour on a stem. It may be benign (not cancerous) or malignant (cancerous).

Pouch An external bag that collects the discharge from a stoma.

Prebiotics Dietary fibre that promotes the growth of 'good' bacteria.

Probiotics 'Good' bacteria.

Prophylaxsis (n), prophylactic (adj.) Treatment taken to avoid disease.

Rectum Short tube that holds faeces until it is ready to be expelled from the anus.

Reflux When stomach contents backflow into the oesophagus.

Sigmoid colon A section of the large bowel on the left side in and near the pelvis.

Sigmoidoscope A medical instrument used for examining the large bowel as far as the sigmoid.

Sign A visible physical change that indicates presence of illness or disease.

Small intestine The small bowel.

Sorbitol A non-sugar sweetener found in some chewing gum.

Sphincter A valve (usually a band of muscle around the gut whch contracts and stops the flow of fluid).

Stenosis Narrowing of tubular structure.

Stricture Localised constriction of tubular structure.

Stoma A surgically created opening.

Stool Another word for faeces.

Symptom A change noticed by the patient that might indicate an ailment.

Total parenteral nutrition (TPN) Fluid nutrients given directly into a vein.

Toxic megacolon Complication of the bowel that causes the colon to dilate.

Ulcer Open sore; hole in a mucous membrane of an internal organ.

Ulcerative colitis A chronic inflammatory disease of the colon.

Villi Small finger-like protrusions in the small intestine that absorb nutrients into the bloodstream.

Visceral Relating to an organ.

Waterbrash An excessive amount of saliva forming in the mouth usually just prior to vomiting.

Xerostomia Dry mouth.

Index

Note: Page numbers in italics indicate figures. Numbers which form prefixes in chemical names have been ignored in filing: e.g. 6-mercaptoprurine files under 'm'.
GIT = gastrointestinal tract; IBD = inflammatory bowel disease; IBS = irritable bowel syndrome

hospitalisation for treatment
of 45; in the oesophagus 62;
in the small intestine 62
odynophagia 125, 133
oesophageal spasm 136
oesophagitis 122, 125, 126,
130, 137, 139
oesophagus: blockages as a
cause of hiccups 62; cancer
in 123, 129, 131, 139, 141;
overview of 3–4; as part of
the gastrointestinal tract 1;
sphincter between stomach
and 122
oils 13
omega-3, 206
omeprazole 115
opiate painkillers 183
oral candidiasis (thrush)
60-61
oral contraceptives 47, 186
organ tension 42, 44
osmotic laxatives 91
osteopaenic bone disease 165,
184
osteoporosis 104, 153, 155,
160, 180
ostomy 207, 260
ostomy surgery 266–7, 272
ovaries 44

pain 41–4, 104, 125, 155,
180
pain receptors 41
painkillers 40, 41, 49, 183,
230, 233
pancolitis 212
pancreas 7, 8, 44, 113

pancreatitis 80, 113
pantoprazole 115
parasites 52, 64
parietal pain 41
Parkinson's disease,
medication for 49, 134
parotid 3
partial bowel resection 208
'passing wind', 55
pectin 87
pepsin 102–3, 122
peptic ulcer disease: bleeding
and perforation 107; causes
of 5, 101–5, 118; complications if untreated 106;
detecting ulcers 28, 31–2;
diagnosis 109–11, 136, 159;
dietary considerations 115,
117; diseases associated with
108–9; diseases with similar
symptoms 112–13; effect of
lifestyle on 116; gastric
ulcers 118; genetic factors
105–6; journals on 289;
nausea caused by ulcers 65;
obstructions caused by
ulcers 107–8; peptic ulcers
102, 118; prognosis
116–17; risk of anaemia
108; risk of cancer 108;
in severely ill patients 105;
symptoms 106, 136, 159;
tests for 110–11, 136, 159;
treating ulcers 114–16;
types of ulcers 118; ulcers in
the duodenum 101, 104,
106, 118; ulcers in the
stomach 101–4, *102*, 106,